Session 2

When I Worry

Sometimes it can be hard to think about what makes us feel worried. Together with your mom or dad, think about what things make you worry or feel nervous. Then, look at the **Everybody Worries Sometimes** worksheet on the next page. Maybe you'll find something you worry about on that list. Feel free to add worries if you do not see them. Remember, *everybody* worries sometimes, even adults.

After you read the list, decide with your mom or dad what kinds of worries you have. Pay special attention to the worries that interfere the most. In other words, which worries prevent you from making friends, learning at school, going places, or getting along with your family? Circle the worries. Highlight the five worries that get in your way the most.

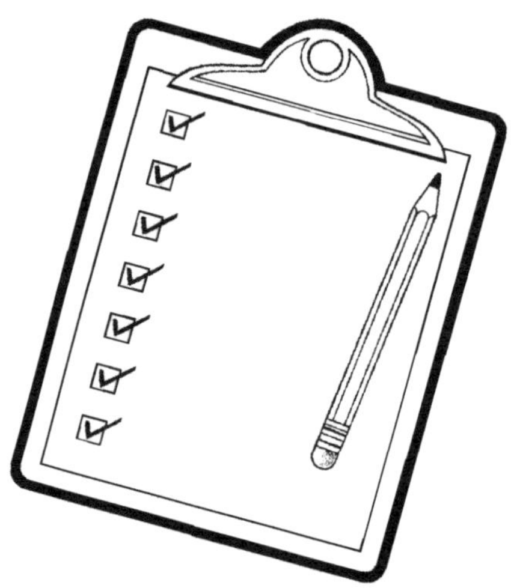

Everybody Worries Sometimes

Kids *and* adults worry.

People worry about. . .

- ☐ Storms and/or tornados
- ☐ Dogs and/or cats
- ☐ Letting go of past events
- ☐ Being late
- ☐ Bugs, spiders, and/or bees
- ☐ The dark
- ☐ Getting to sleep
- ☐ Talking to new people
- ☐ Being away from family
- ☐ Being home alone
- ☐ Using public bathrooms
- ☐ Getting a disease
- ☐ Making mistakes
- ☐ Going to someone's house
- ☐ Starting homework
- ☐ Trying new foods
- ☐ Getting to sleep on my own
- ☐ ____________________
- ☐ ____________________
- ☐ Being in a room by myself
- ☐ World events
- ☐ Being teased
- ☐ Loud noises
- ☐ Heights
- ☐ Starting a conversation
- ☐ Parents going out
- ☐ Germs
- ☐ Asking for help
- ☐ Dying
- ☐ Getting lost
- ☐ Scary movies
- ☐ Lots of people
- ☐ Talking in school
- ☐ Changes
- ☐ Performing in front of others

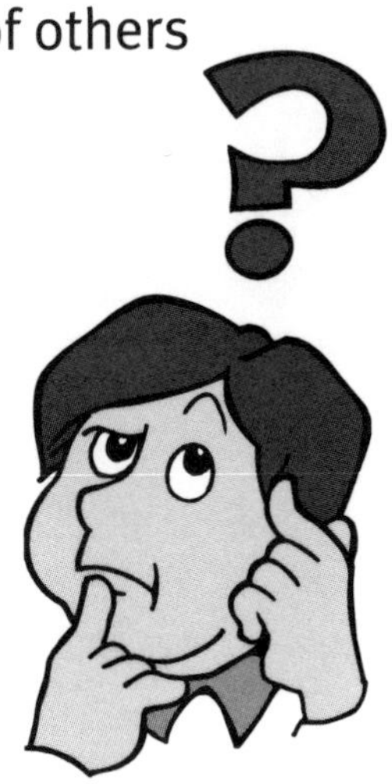

Do you worry about any of these things?
Think about how much these worries bother you each day.

Kids do different things when they get worried. Some kids get really quiet. Other kids get restless and have a hard time sitting still. Sometimes, it's hard to recognize what we do when we get nervous. Together with your mom or dad, think and talk about how your body reacts when you worry or feel nervous.

After talking with your mom or dad, circle on the **How I React When I Worry** worksheet on the next page how your body reacts when you worry. Highlight your five most common reactions to worry.

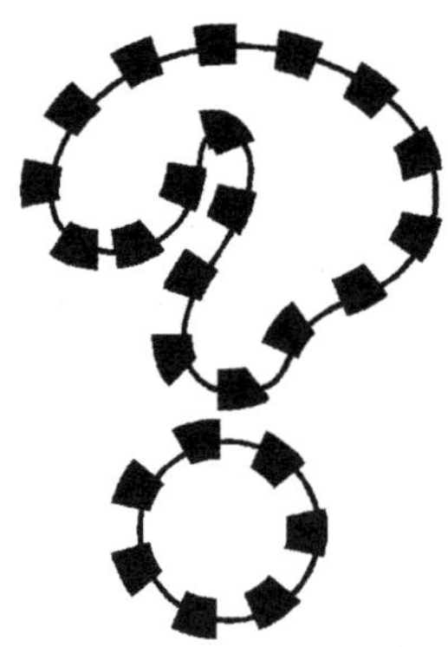

How I React When I Worry

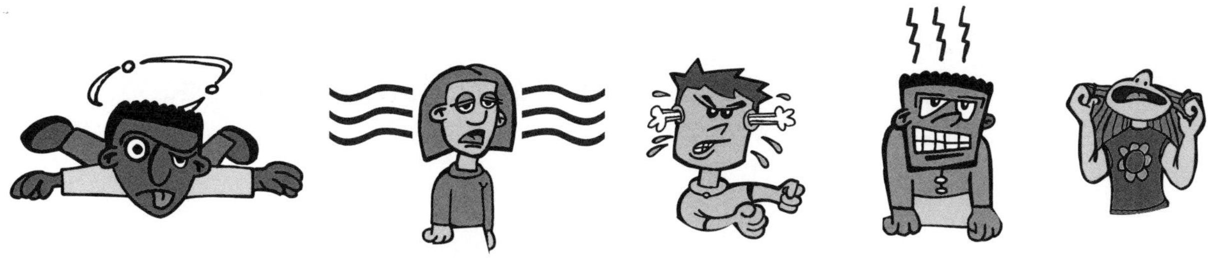

The Many Faces of Anxiety

- ❑ Cry
- ❑ Scream or yell
- ❑ Get quiet
- ❑ Get angry
- ❑ Act silly
- ❑ Have trouble sitting still
- ❑ Feel sick
- ❑ Hit somebody
- ❑ Blush
- ❑ Get sweaty palms
- ❑ Resist or refuse to do something
- ❑ ______________________________
- ❑ ______________________________
- ❑ ______________________________
- ❑ Cough
- ❑ Get a dry mouth
- ❑ Get a stomachache
- ❑ Get a headache
- ❑ Feel like my muscles get tense
- ❑ Laugh
- ❑ Get itchy skin
- ❑ Feel like my heart races
- ❑ Breathe fast
- ❑ Get goose bumps
- ❑ Put my head down

On the next page, draw a picture of what you look like when you worry. Talk with your mom or dad, and look at the list you just made about what you do when you worry. This will help you to think about how to draw your picture.

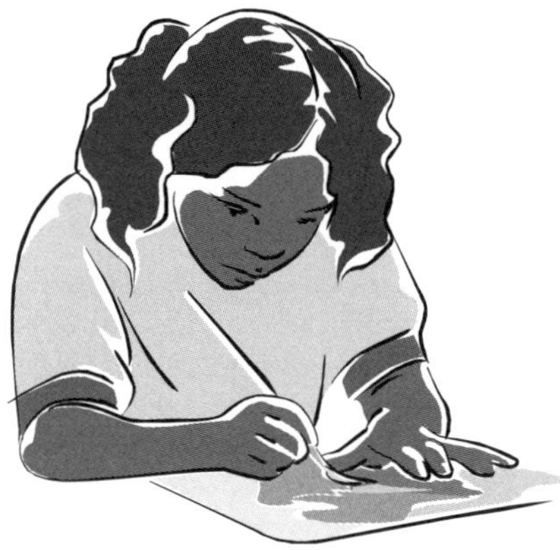

This Is What I Look Like When I Worry

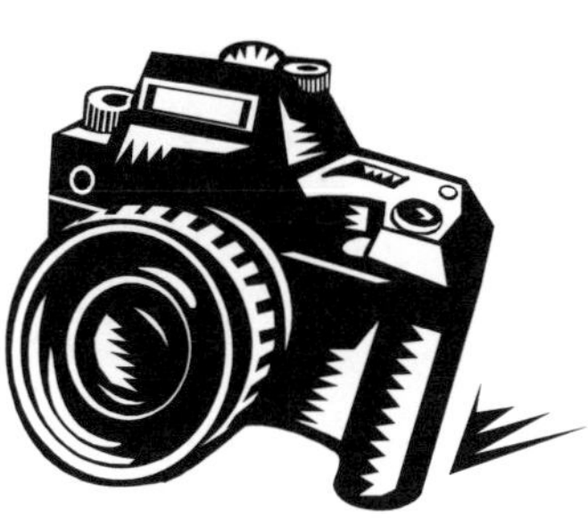

Session 3

Time Spent Worrying

Now you are going to look at how much time you spend worrying during the day.

On the next pages, you are going to read about Michael, Annie, and John. They are kids your age who spend time worrying during the day. One of them worries a lot, one of them worries sometimes, and one of them does not spend much time worrying at all.

Together with your mom or dad, figure out how much time they each spend worrying.

After you read about Michael, Annie, and John, you are going to see how much time *you* spend worrying *now*. Then, you will predict how much time you think you'll spend worrying in the *future*, once you learn to handle your worry.

Start reading about Michael, Annie, and John on the next pages!

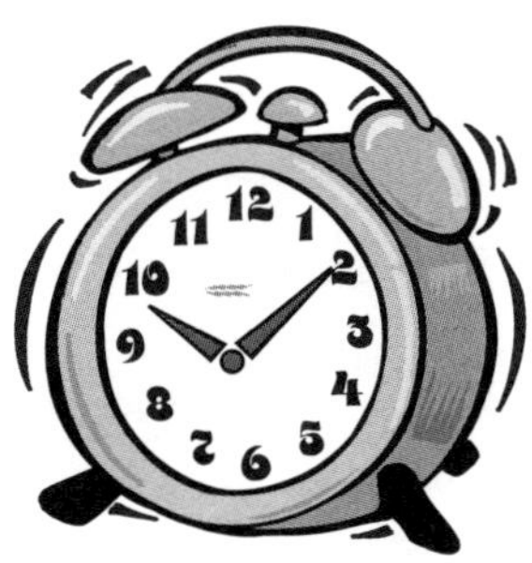

Time Michael Spends Worrying

Michael worries about a lot of different things. He spends a lot of his time during the day worrying!

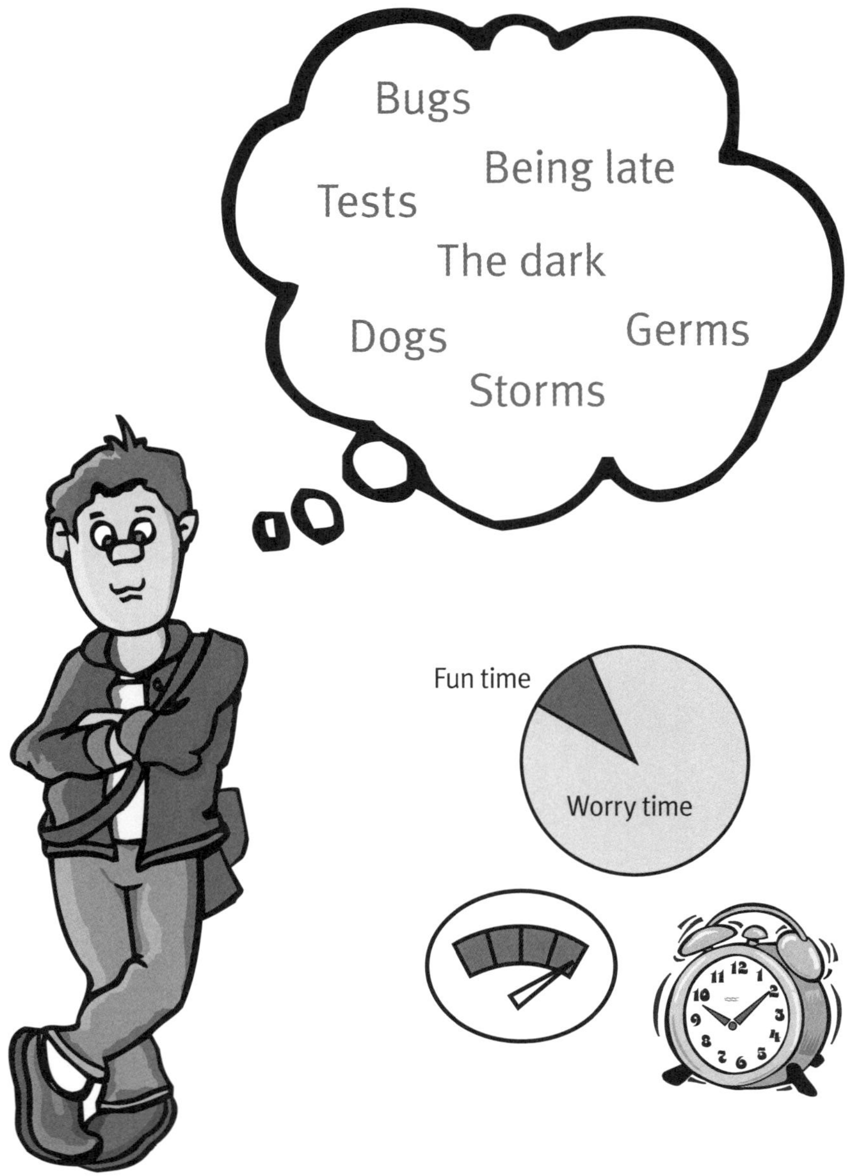

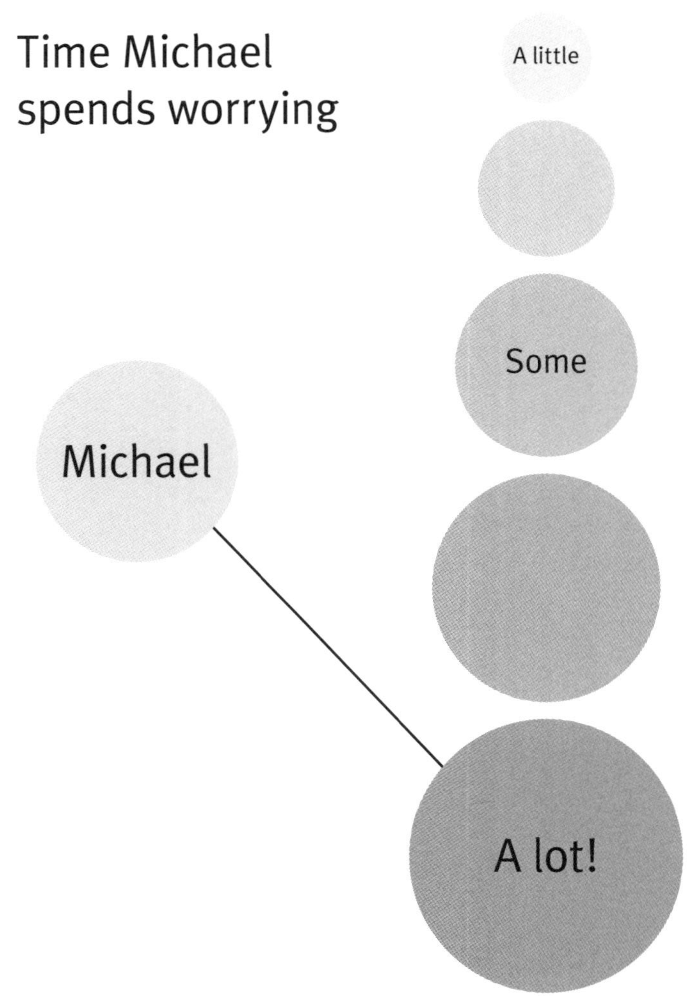

Michael has no time to do anything fun.
He spends almost all of his time worrying!

Time Annie Spends Worrying

Annie sometimes gets nervous about tests, and she is a little scared of big storms.
How much time do you think she spends worrying?

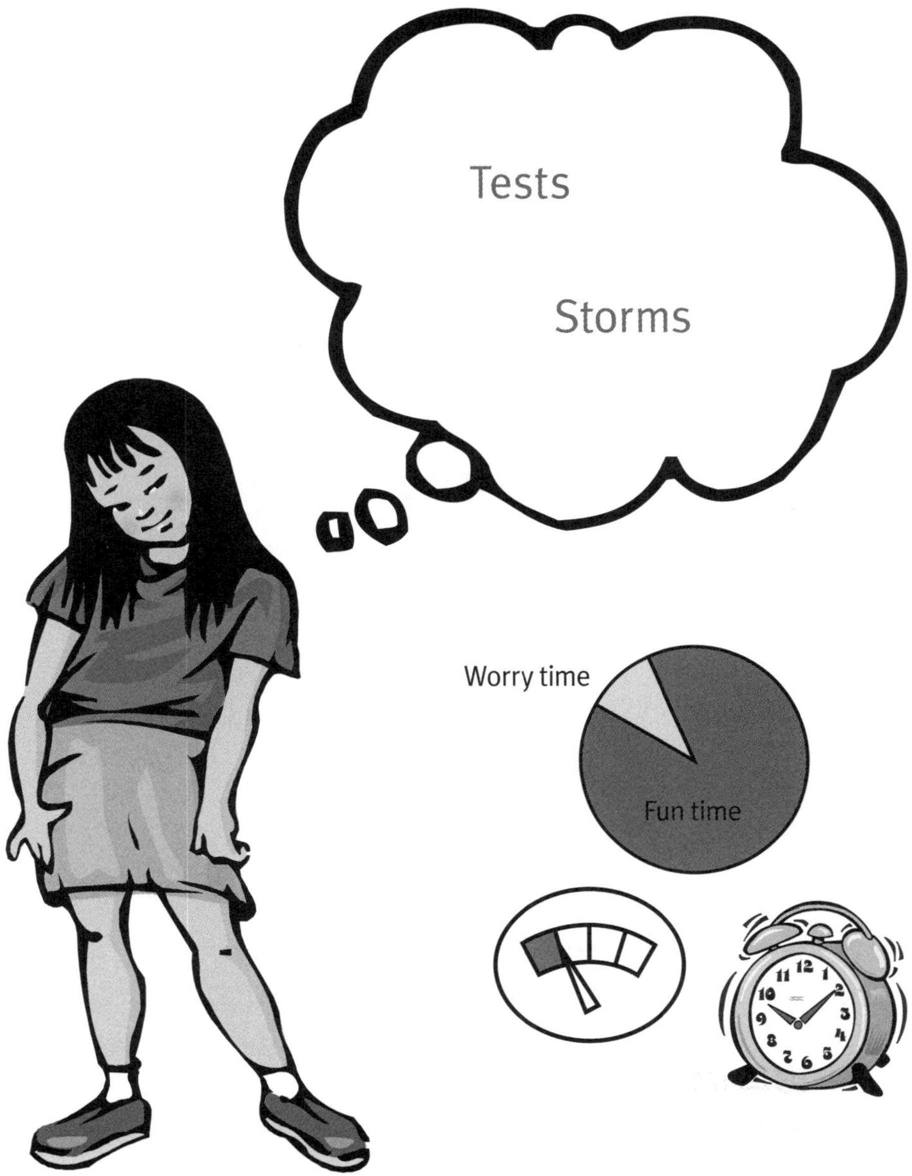

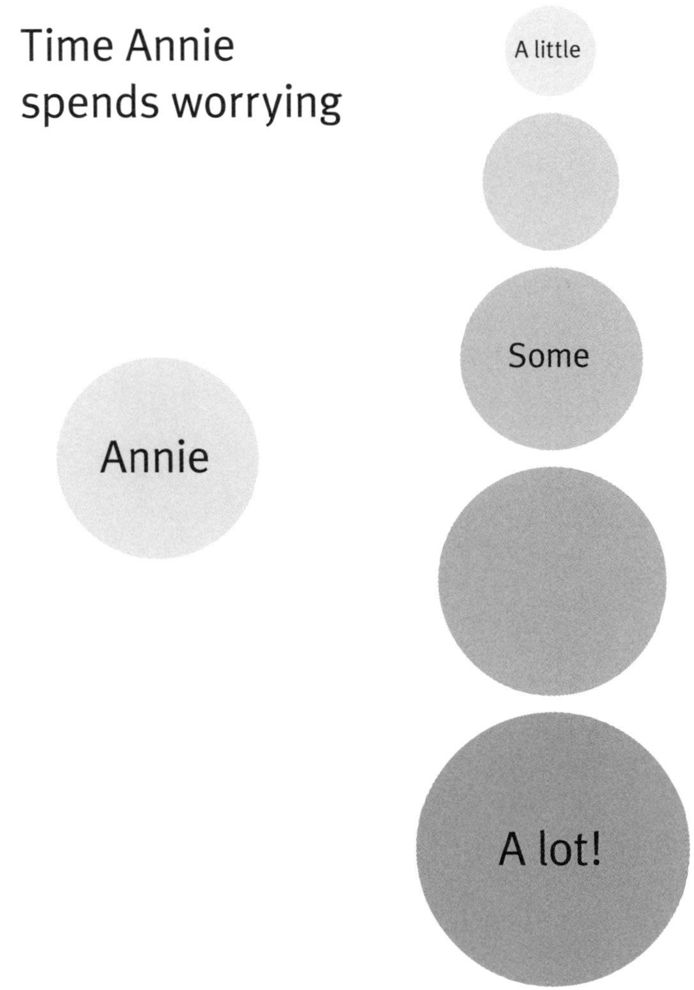

Time John Spends Worrying

John worries about tests, homework, making mistakes, and being late.
How much time do you think he spends worrying?

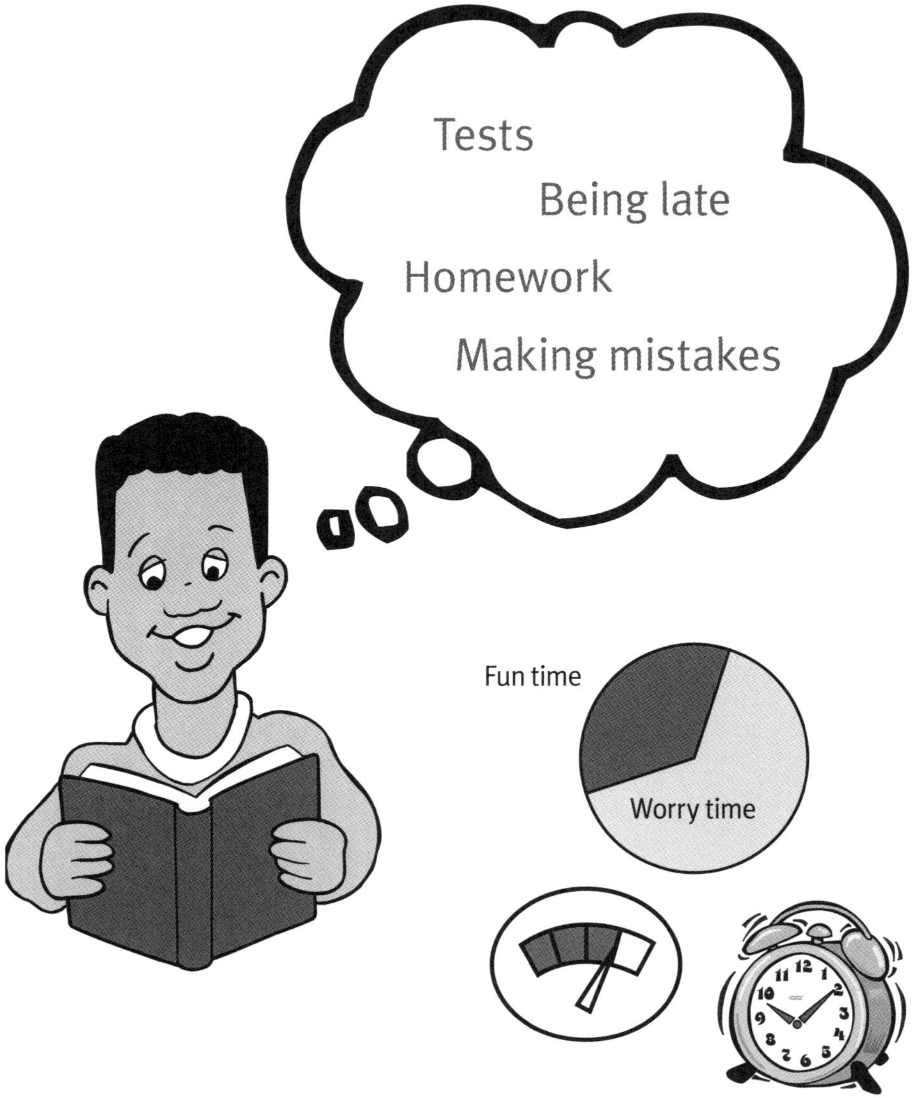

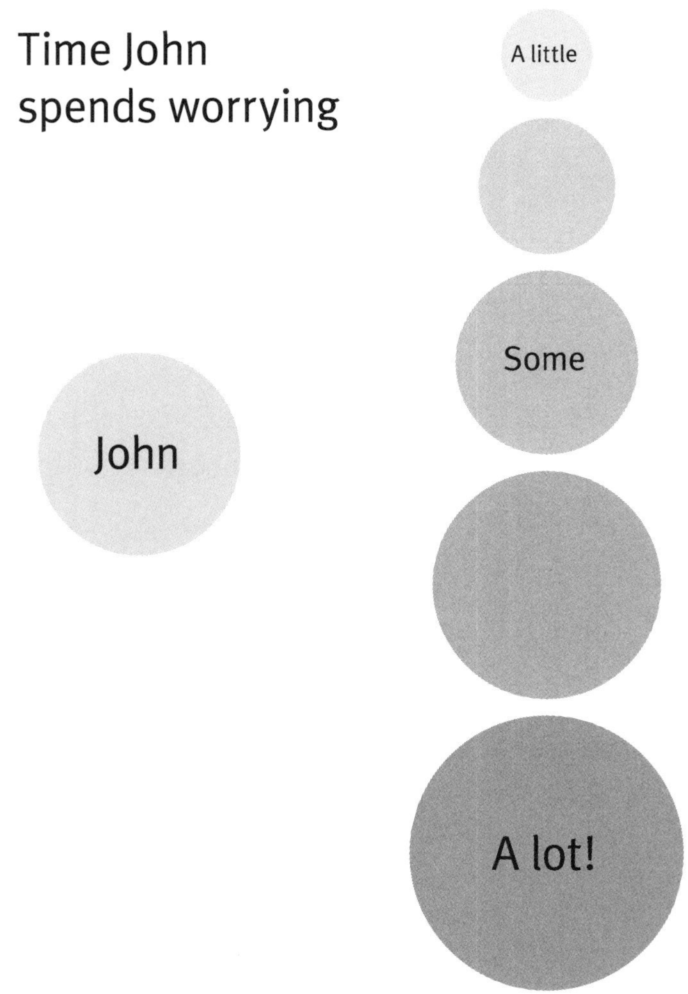

How Much Time Do You Spend Worrying Now?

Write down your worries here!

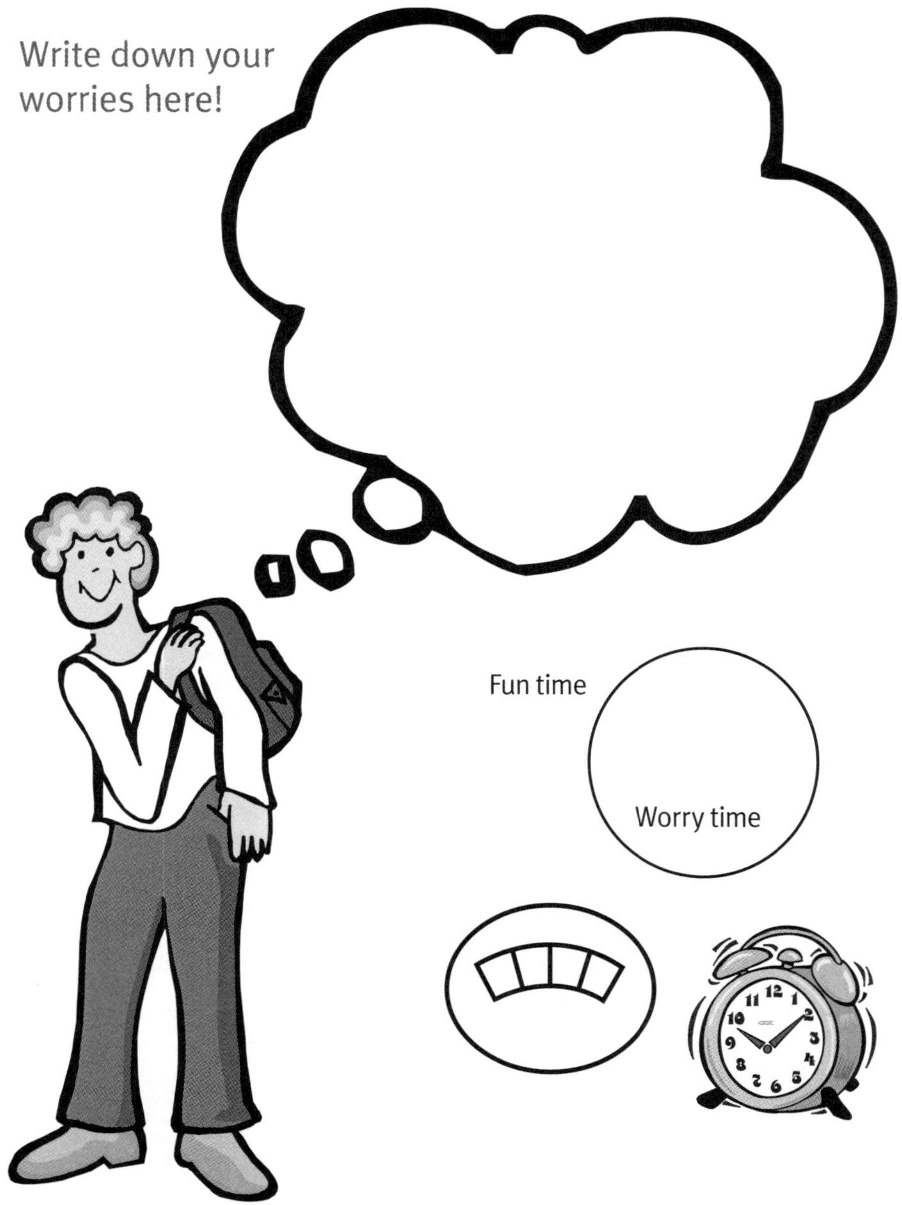

Time I spend worrying

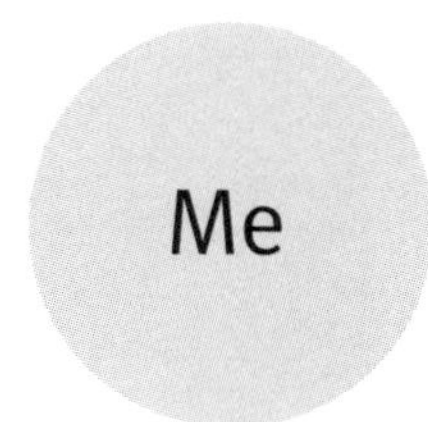

How Much Time Do You Predict You Will Spend Worrying in the Future?

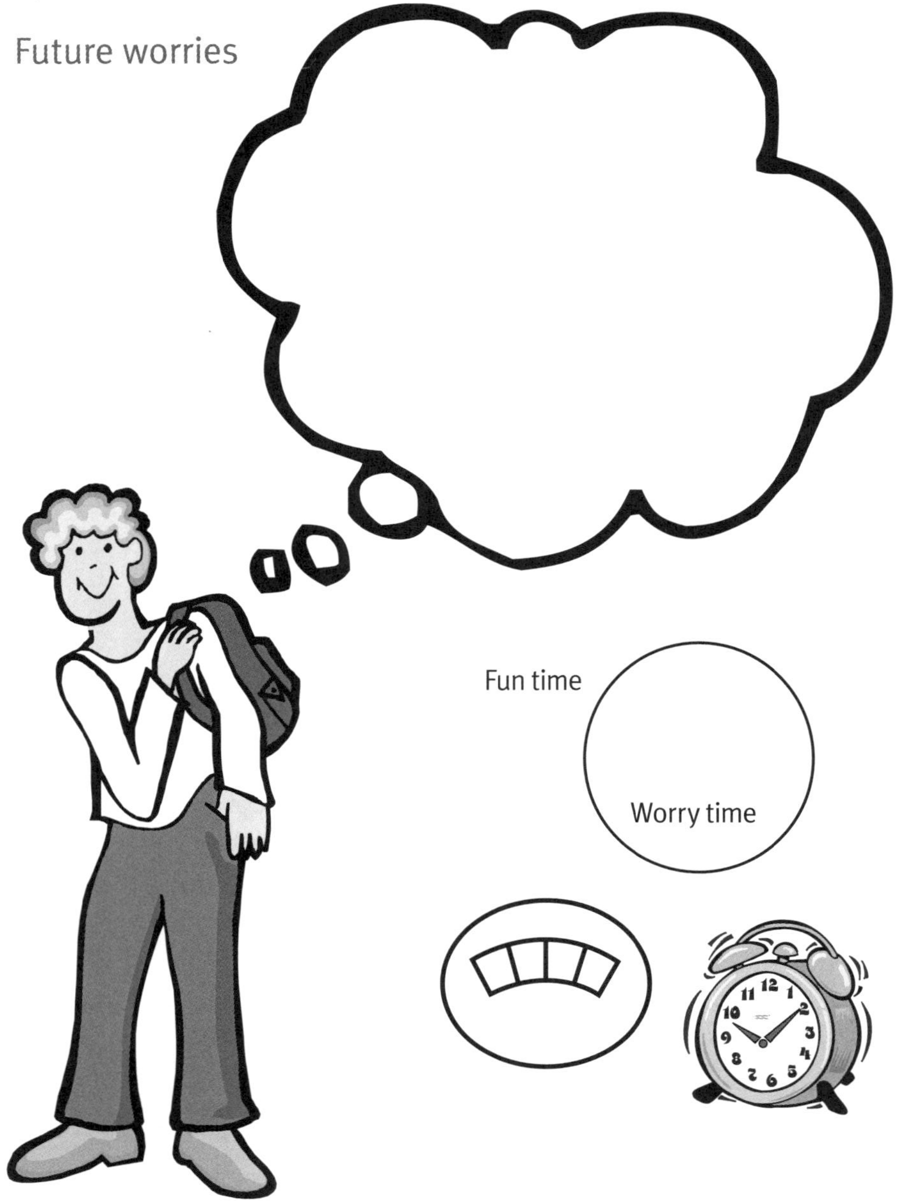

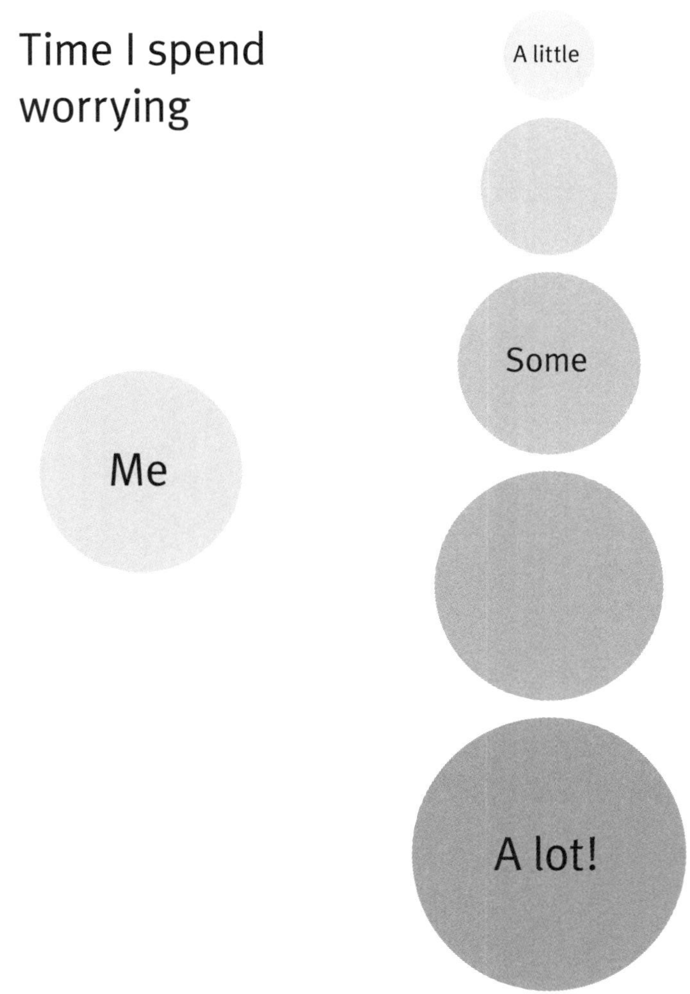

When Worry Goes Away, I'll...

Write what you will spend your time doing
in the future when you no longer worry as much.

1. ______________________________
2. ______________________________
3. ______________________________
4. ______________________________
5. ______________________________

Or draw!

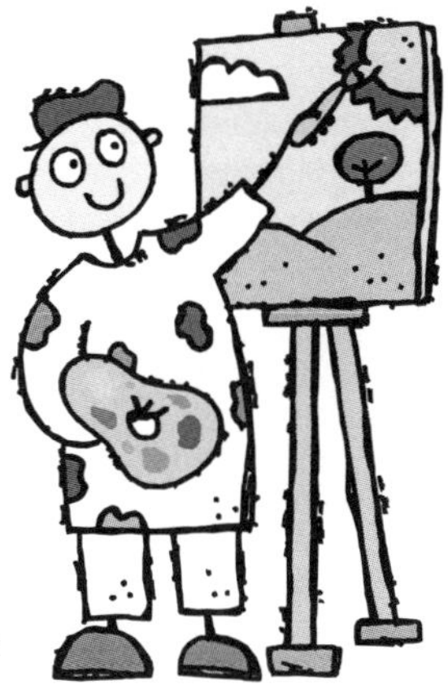

Next, you are going to create several characters. Your first character is your WORRY BUG. Almost everyone has a worry bug. Worry bugs are the fears and anxiety that get in our way and make it hard for us to learn in school, have fun at home, or play with friends.

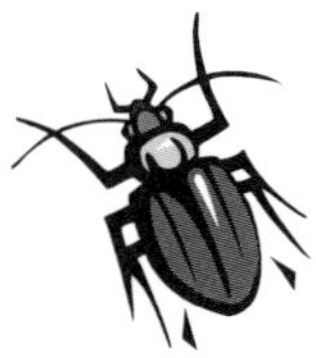

What does your worry bug look like?
What will you call it?

Once you have drawn or created your worry bug on the next page, draw or create your HELPER BUG. A helper bug is an imaginary creature that helps you defeat your worry bug!

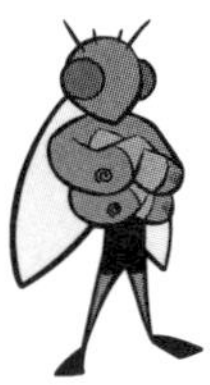

What does your helper bug look like?
What will you call it?

Next, write the names of all of the friends, family members, or fictional characters that can help you beat worry!

Finally, create something (either with Play-Doh or markers) that shows you and your helper bug squashing your worry bug!

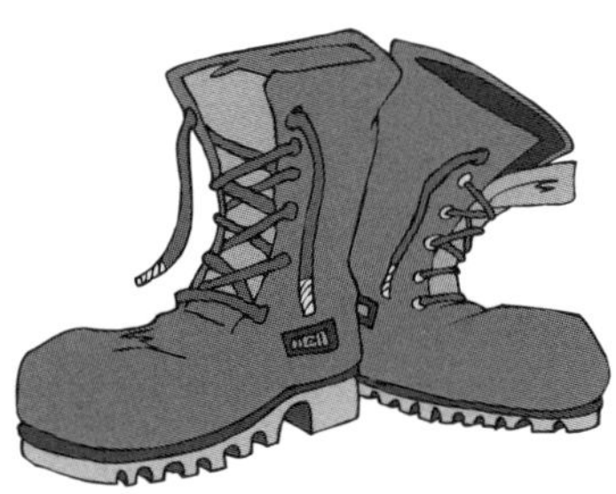

My Worry Bug

Its name is ______________________________

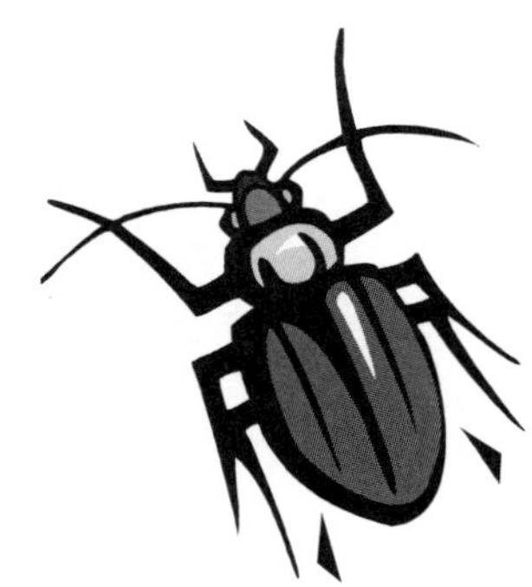

My Helper Bug

Its name is ______________________________

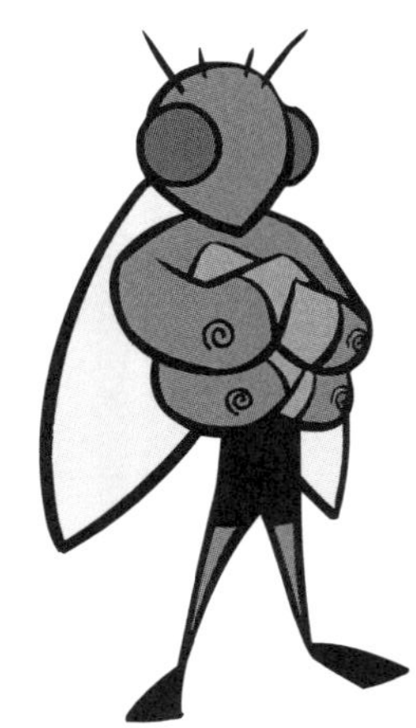

My Team to Help Beat Worry

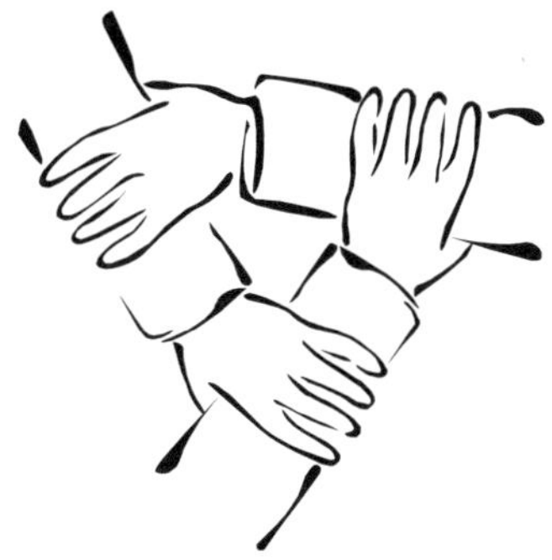

Squashing My Worry Bug!

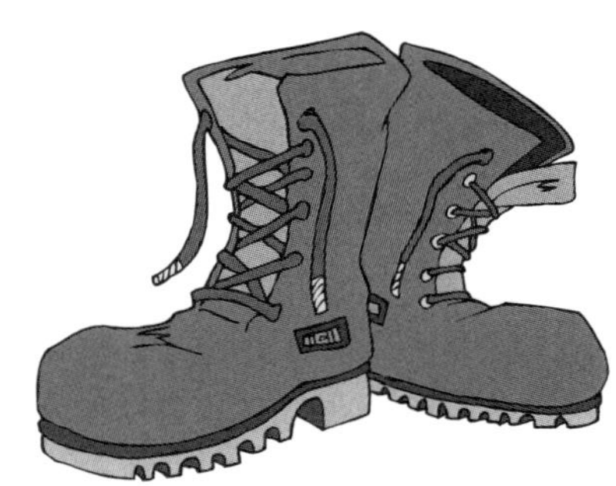

Session 4

What Worry Does to My Body

Beginning to Measure Worry

On the picture on the **What Worry Does to Your Body** worksheet on the next page, circle or color how worry makes *your* body feel. For example, if worrying makes your stomach upset, circle or color the butterflies on the boy's stomach.

What does worry do to your body?

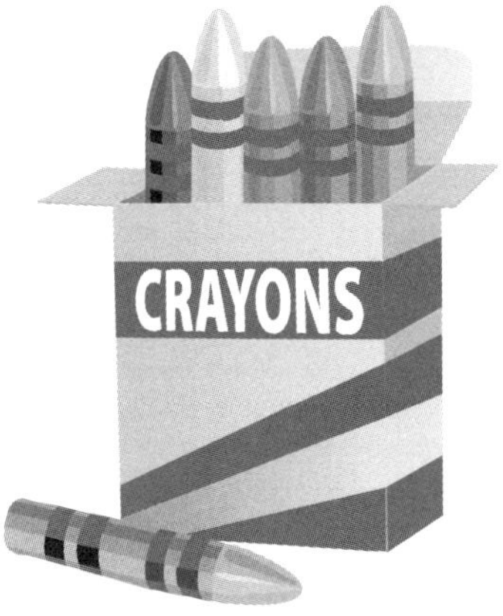

What Worry Does to Your Body

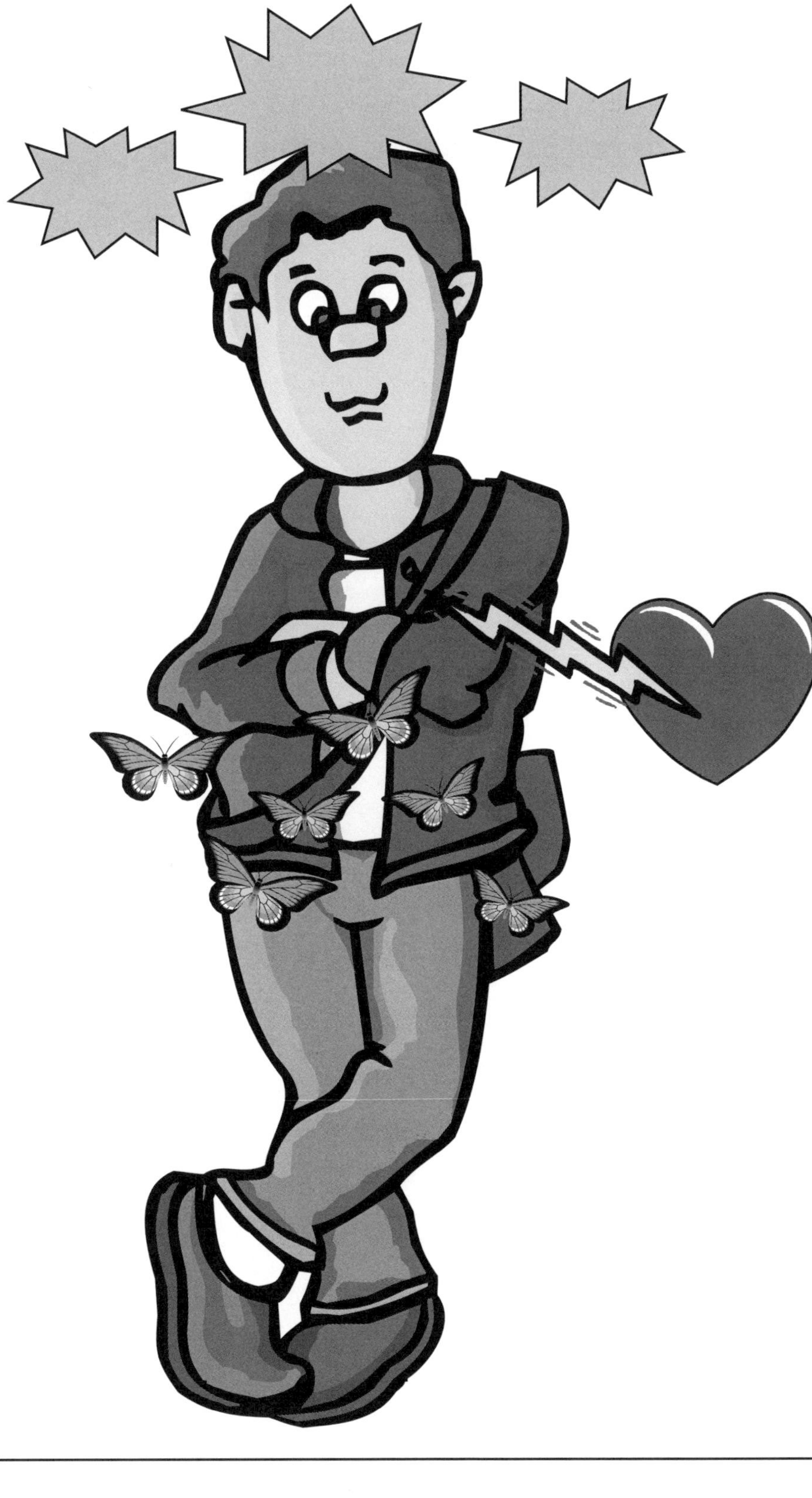

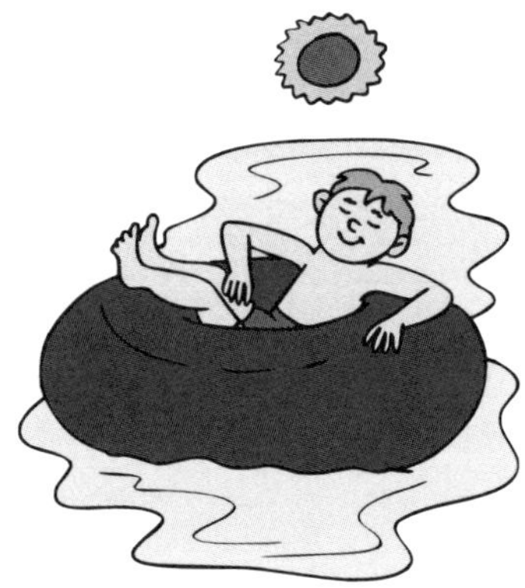

We just practiced deep breathing to help our body's reaction to worry. Using the list on the next page as a guideline, think about what else you can do to help your body relax. How can you help your body feel better so you can think and make a plan to handle your worry?

What do you like to do to relax?

Circle your favorite activities on the following page.

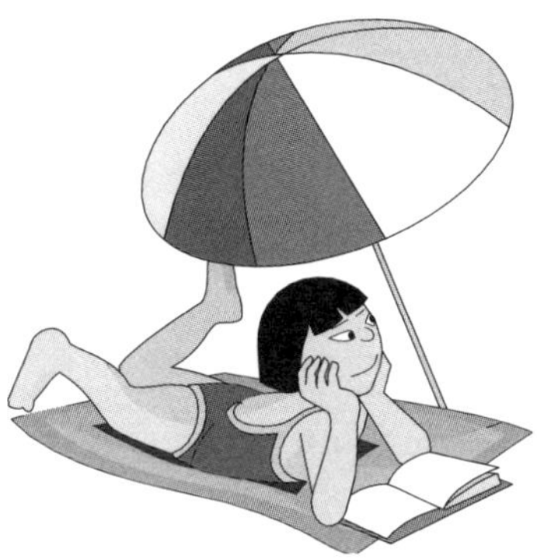

If your favorite activities are not on the list, write them down! Figure out when you'll do these activities, and write them in on the **Schedule for Calming and/or Relaxing Activities.**

Post these pages in your house so that you can remember to relax every day!

What I Like to Do to Relax

Listen to music

Play with my pet

Read a book

Go for a walk

Jump on the trampoline

Play a sport

Ride a bike

Watch television

Play video games

Play with and/or collect trading cards

Play my musical instrument

Take a warm bath

Snuggle up with pillows

Sit quietly

Sing

Cook

Draw pictures

Talk with a friend

Write in a journal

Squeeze a Koosh ball

What else?

____

____

____

____

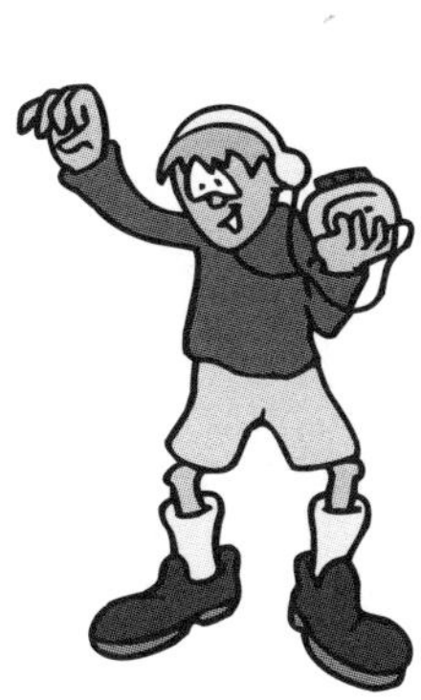

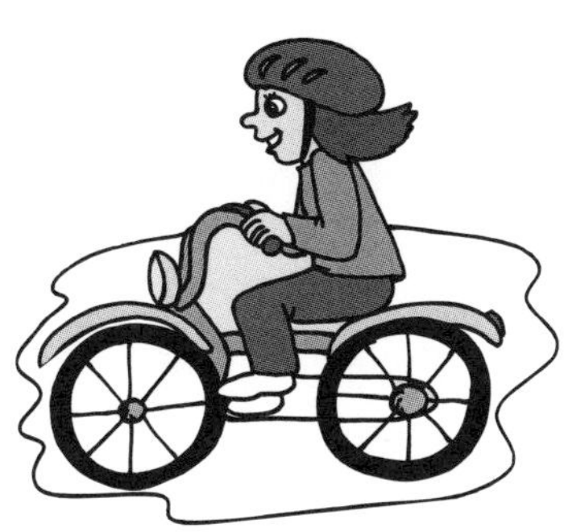

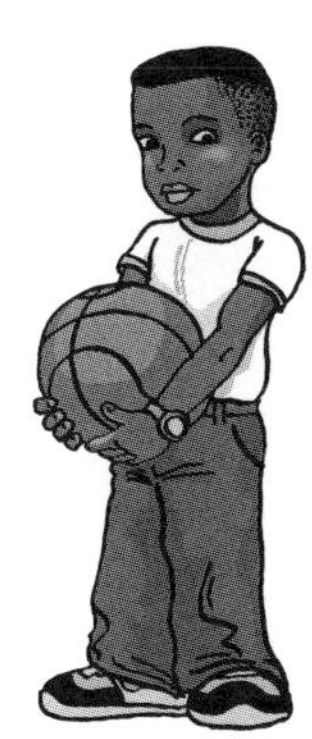

Schedule for Calming and/or Relaxing Activities

Calming Activities	Sunday	Monday	Tuesday	Wednesday	Thursday	Friday	Saturday
1.							
2.							
3.							
4.							
5.							
6.							
7.							
8.							

Reward Plan:

Completing 1–2 activities per week = ____________________

Completing 3–4 activities per week = ____________________

Completing 5–6+ activities per week = ____________________

On the next page, look at the list of worries and fears with your mom or dad.

Which ones do you worry about sometimes?
Which ones do you worry about a lot?
Which ones do you never worry about?

Most important, select the fears or worries that get in your way. If you want to, you can add other fears and/or worries in the blanks on your checklist.

Next, think about where you would be on your stress-o-meter if faced with one of your worry situations.
Write the number next to the worry.

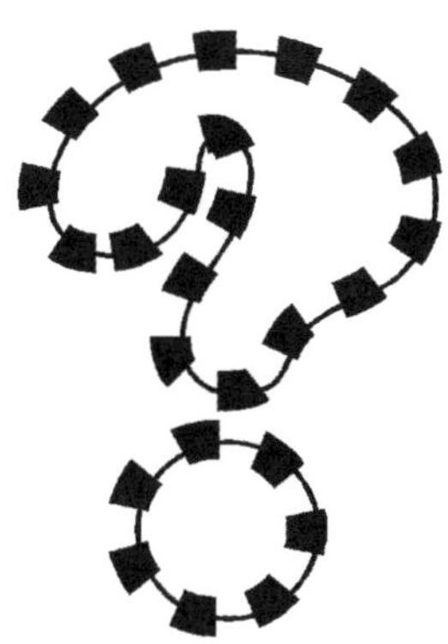

My Checklist of Fears, Worries, and Irritations

I'm afraid of, worried about, or irritated about . . .

	No	Sometimes	A lot	Stress-o-meter rating (1–8)
Being late				
Being home alone				
Making mistakes				
The dark				
Letting go of past events				
Dogs and/or cats				
Storms and/or tornados				
Bugs, spiders, and/or bees				
Getting a disease				
Being teased				
Germs				
Trying new foods				
Being away from family				
Using public bathrooms				
Talking to new people				
Talking in school				
Getting to sleep				
Scary movies				
Changes				
Asking for help				
Parents going out				
Getting lost				
Dying				
Starting homework				
World events				
Going to someone's house				
Loud noises				
Heights				
Starting a conversation				
Being in a room by myself				
Performing in front of others				
Other:				

Session 5

The Mind–Body Connection

Steps to Success: Finding My Target

Biggest worry

Pretty big worry

Medium worry

Bit of a worry

Not much of a worry

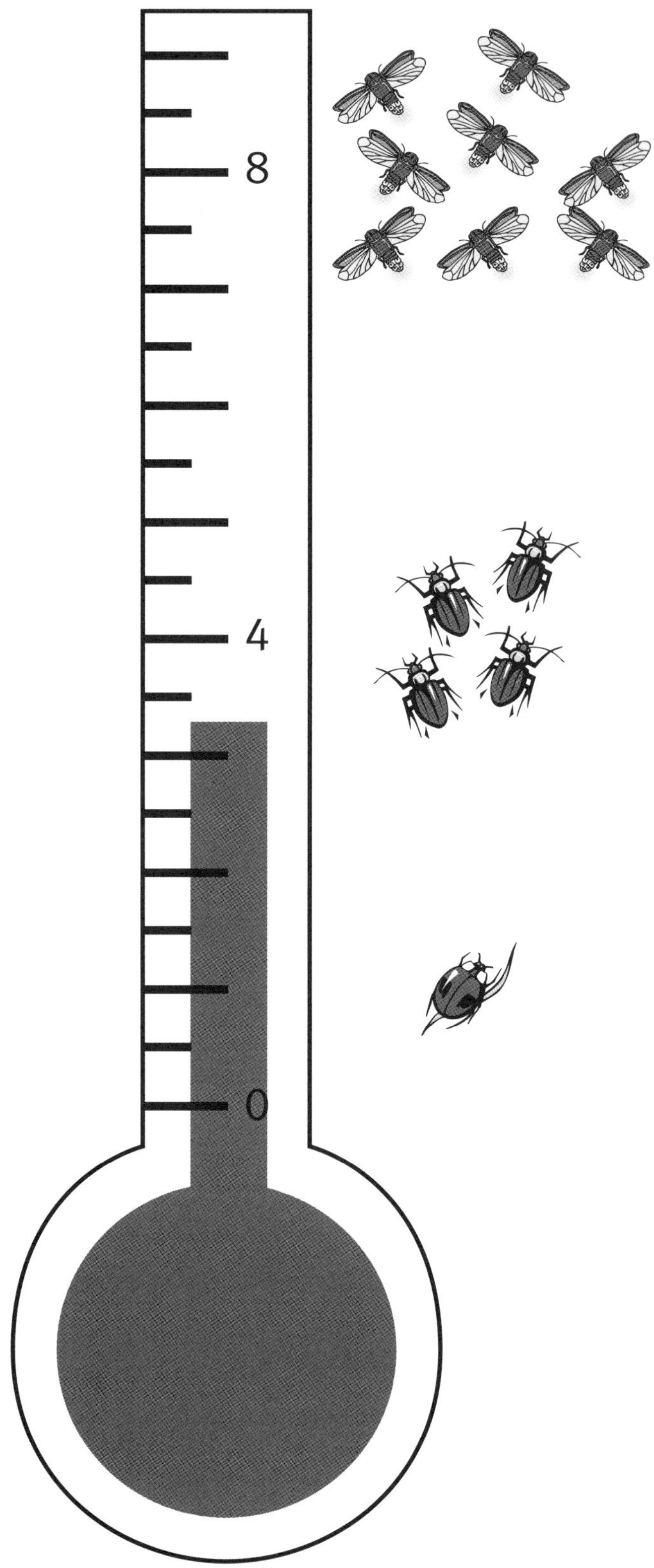

Fear Tracker

Identify up to five fears and/or worries that get in your way. Using your stress-o-meter, please rate on a scale of 1–8 (with *1* meaning *not much of a worry* and *8* meaning *the biggest worry*) the level of stress and/or anxiety you experience when faced with each fear.

Fears	Week 5		Week 6		Week 7		Week 8		Week 9		Week 10	
	Parent	Child	Parent	Child	Parent	Child	Parent	Child	Parent	Child	Parent	Child
1.												
2.												
3.												
4.												
5.												

Fears	Week 11		Week 12		Week 13		Week 14		Booster session	
	Parent	Child	Parent	Child	Parent	Child	Parent	Child	Parent	Child
1.										
2.										
3.										
4.										
5.										

On the next page, you will meet Matthew, who is afraid of snakes. When he goes to the zoo and sees a snake, his mind becomes very active, he begins to think a lot about the snake, and he worries about what might happen.

How will Matthew's body feel when he thinks these thoughts?

Take a look and see!

What do you think?

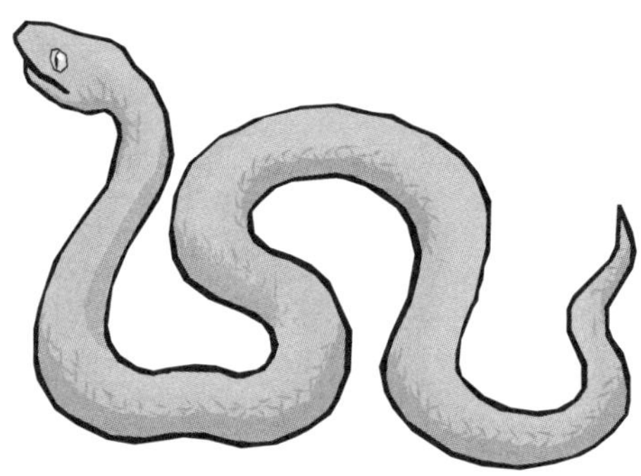

Active Minds

At the zoo one day . . .

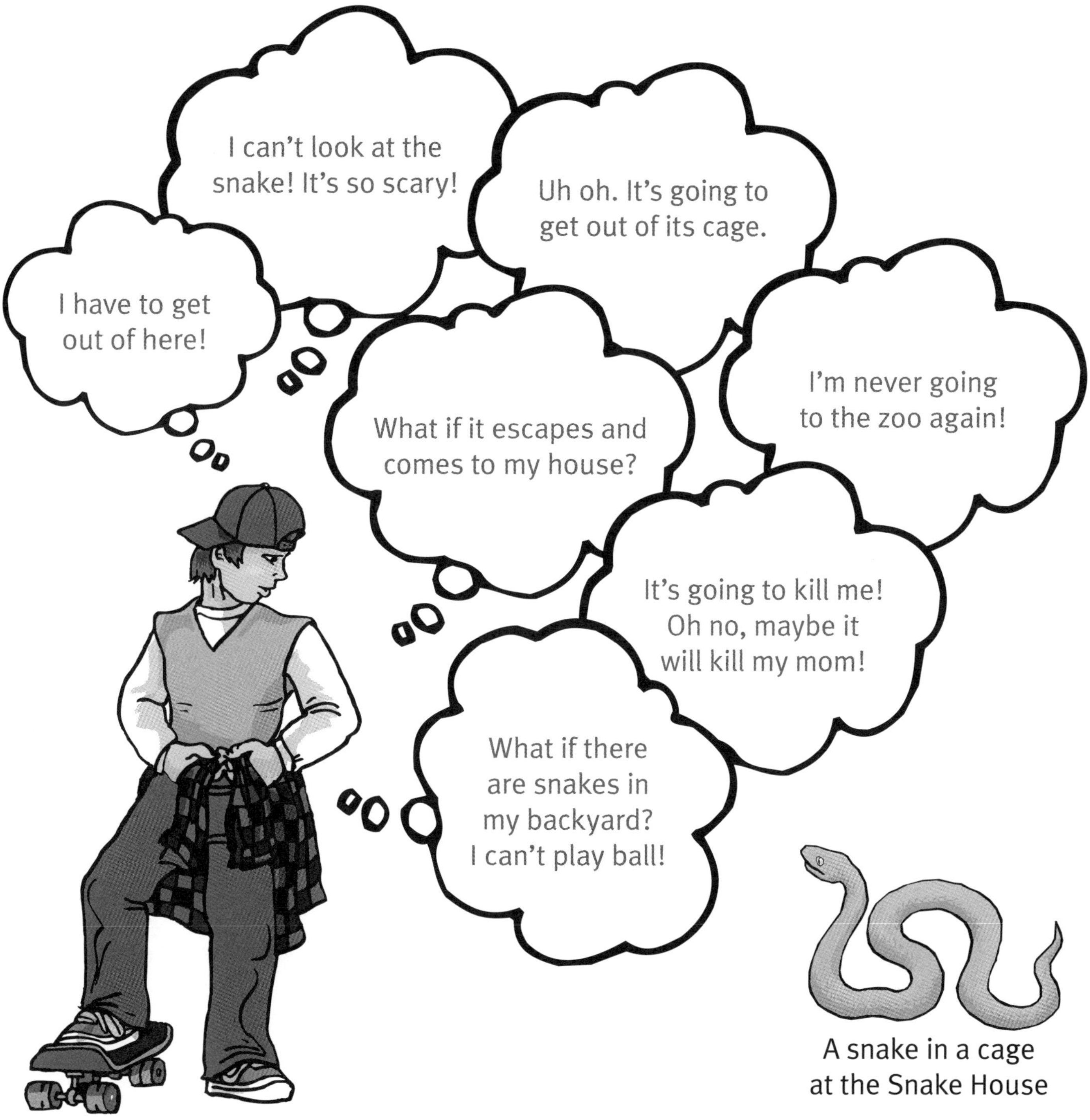

A snake in a cage at the Snake House

Will thinking these thoughts make him feel better or worse?

On the next page, see if you can help Matthew. Write down what Matthew might think or say to help his body feel less anxious when he sees the snake.

How will Matthew's body feel when he thinks these thoughts?

What do you think?

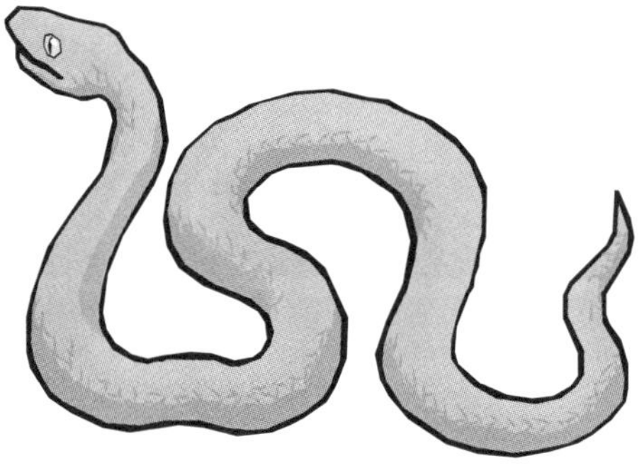

Helpful Thoughts

At the zoo one day . . .

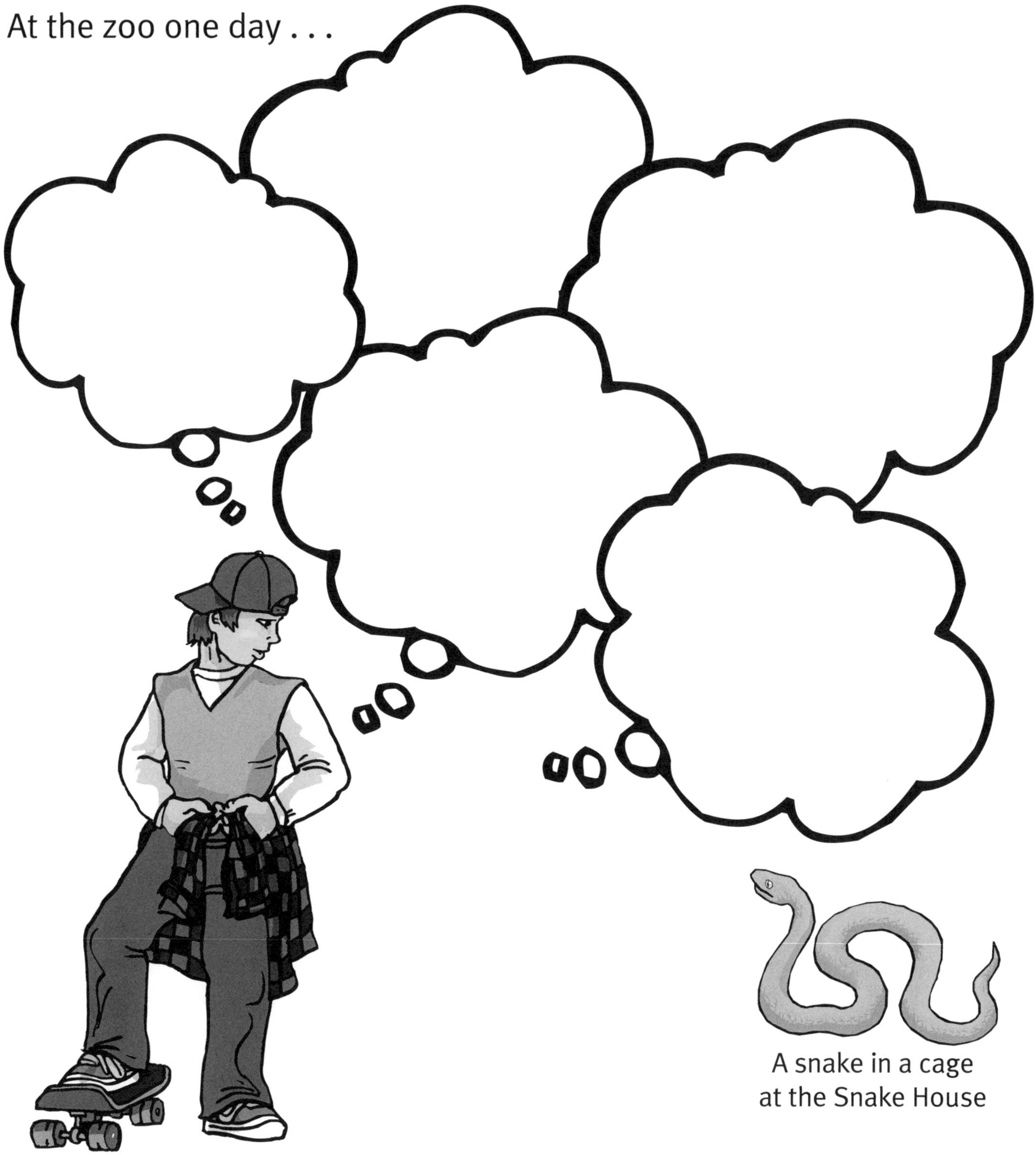

A snake in a cage
at the Snake House

Will thinking these thoughts make him feel better or worse?

Suggestions for Helpful Thoughts

"This is just a 'false alarm.'"

"I can face my fear; nothing bad will happen."

"The worry feelings will go away."

"I can handle this."

"This is no big deal."

"It's my worry bug; I can squash it!"

"I can fight back with facts."

Fight back with facts:

The glass cage is very thick.

Snakes hardly ever escape from cages.

The snake does not know where I live.

Now it's your turn! Think about a situation that makes you feel really anxious or worried. For example, maybe you feel really anxious when you hear thunder.

On the next page, write down the situation in the space at the top of the **Active Minds** worksheet.

Next, think about how your body feels and what happens when your mind becomes active. What does your ACTIVE MIND say? What are you thinking during this situation? Will thinking these thoughts make your body feel better or worse?

Write down how your body feels and what your thoughts are in the thought bubbles.

Active Minds

One day ____

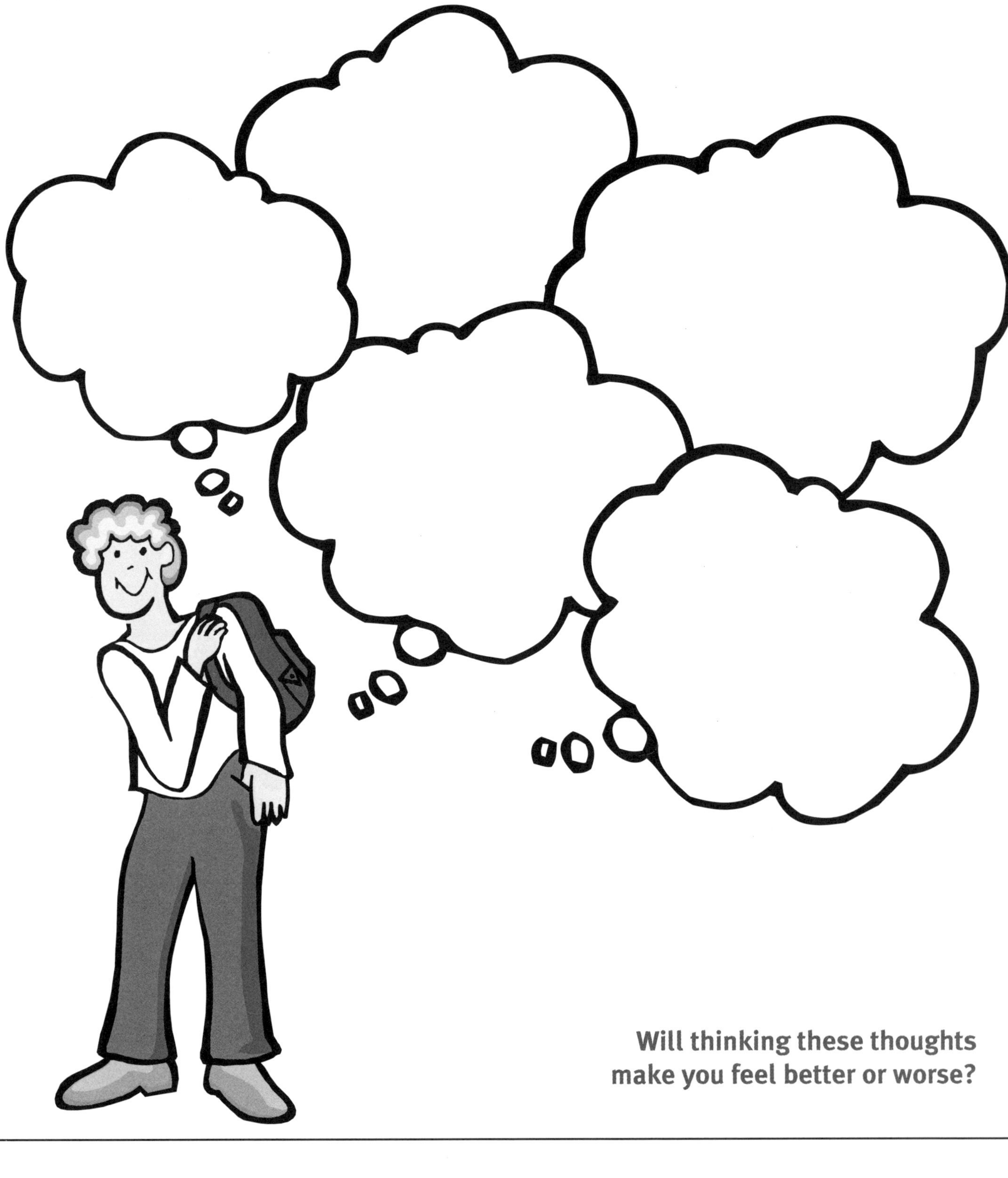

Will thinking these thoughts make you feel better or worse?

Now, think of some helpful thoughts that would make you feel better in this situation.

How will your body feel if you think helpful thoughts?

Write your helpful thoughts down on the next page!

Helpful Thoughts

One day ______________________________

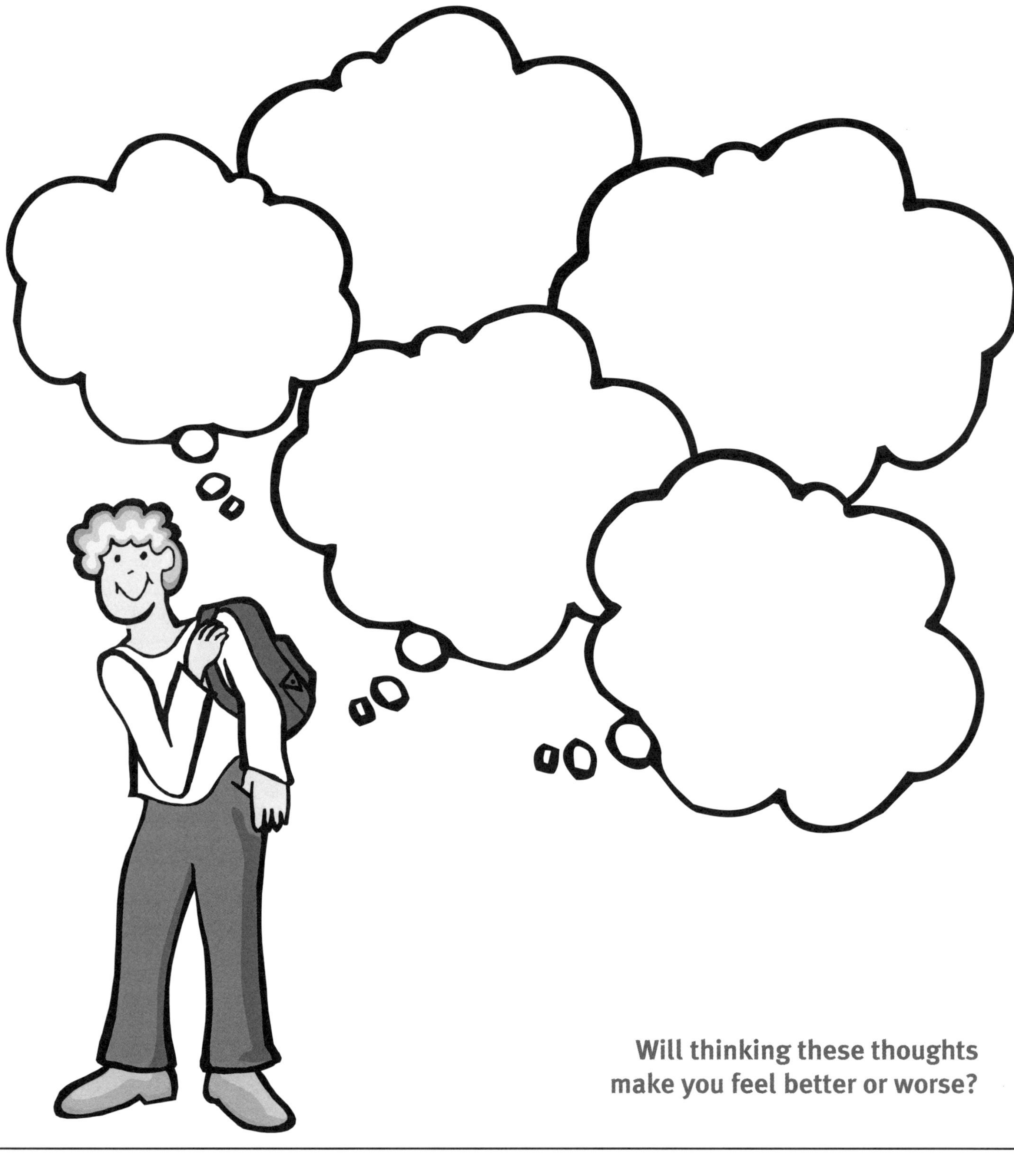

Will thinking these thoughts make you feel better or worse?

Session 6

More Mind–Body Connections

Introduction to Exposure

On the next page, draw a picture of yourself relaxing.

What activity are you doing?
How does your body feel?
What are you thinking?

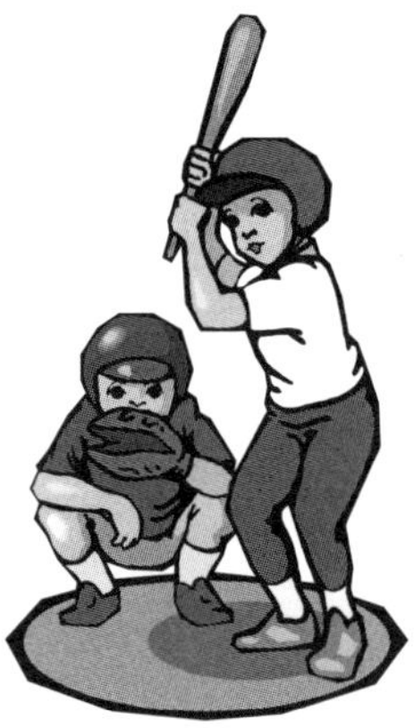

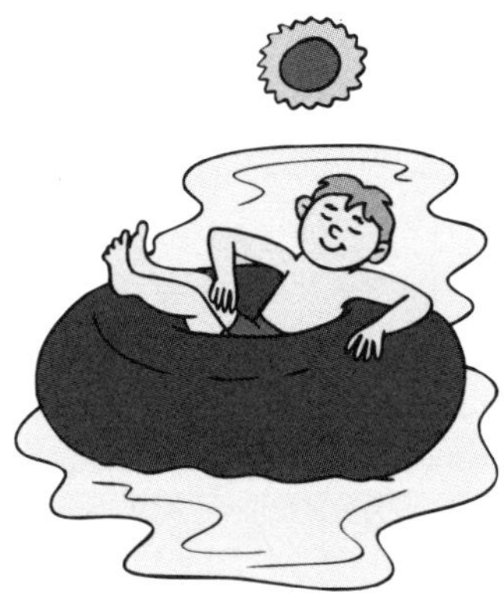

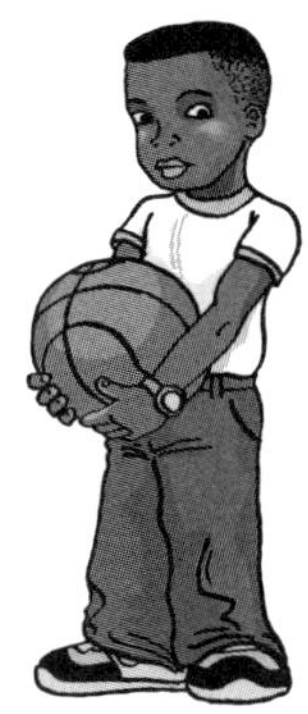

This Is Me Relaxing . . .

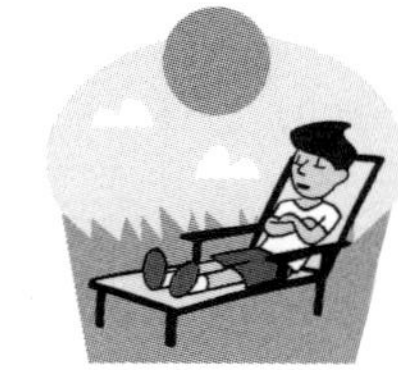

I feel ______________________________ I'm thinking ______________________________

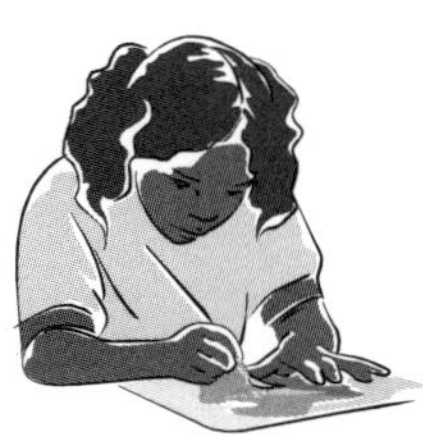

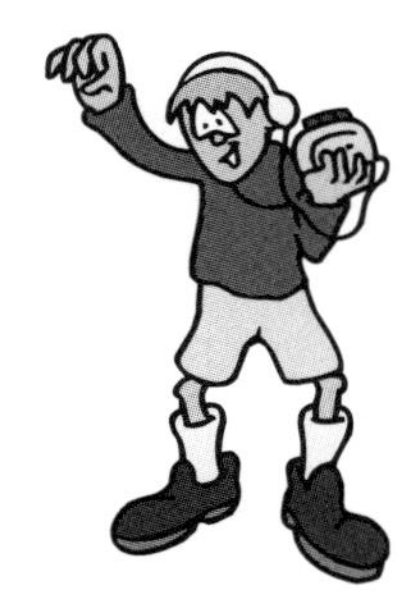

It's time to visit Matthew, the boy who is afraid of snakes, again. On the next page, you will see what happens to Matthew's body when he sees a snake at the zoo. His body alarm goes off, and his mind becomes active.

As Matthew begins to think more worried thoughts, his body alarm goes off even more!

After you read about Matthew, fill in your own **Alarm Chain Reaction** worksheet.

1. Pick a situation that makes you feel worried.

2. Write down how your body feels and what you think when you get worried.

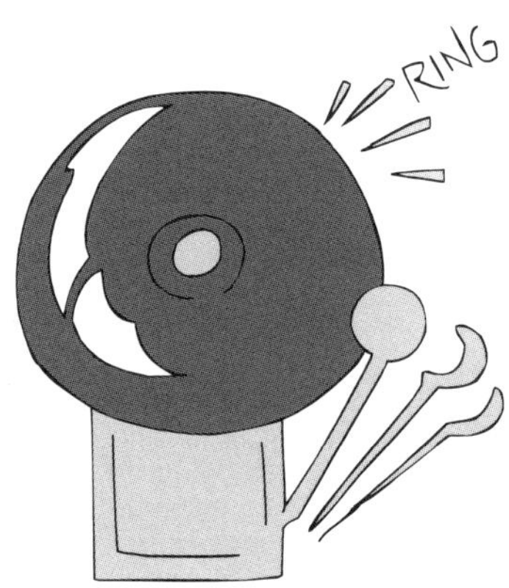

Alarm Chain Reaction

Matthew sees a snake in a cage at the zoo . . .

1

Physical feeling
First, Matthew starts to get butterflies in his stomach.

Thoughts
Oh no, it's a snake.
I don't like snakes!

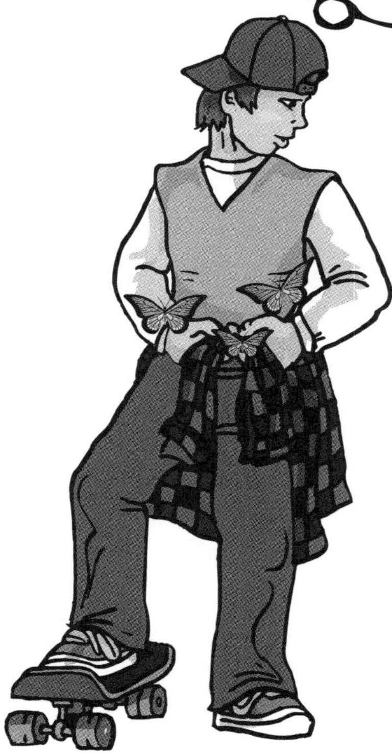

2

Physical feeling
Then, his heart starts beating faster, he gets grouchy, his head starts to hurt, and the butterflies in his stomach get worse.

Thoughts
What if it gets out?!
It might bite me.

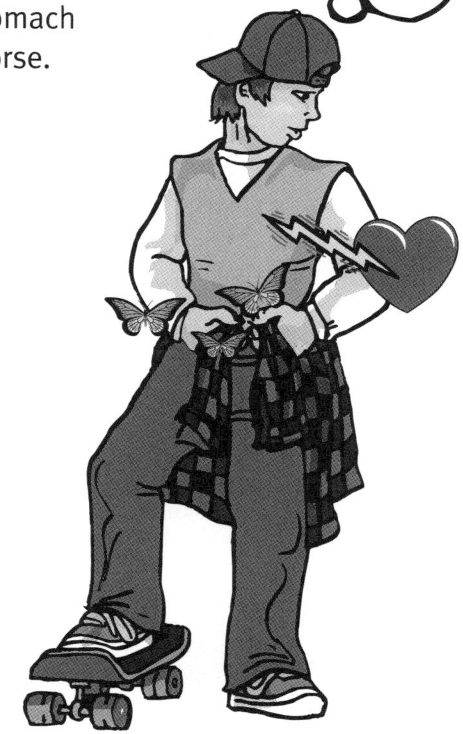

3

Physical feeling
Finally, Matthew becomes so anxious he leaves the zoo. His head really hurts, and he's really upset.

Thoughts
It's coming after me!
I have to get out of here!
I'm never going
to the zoo again!

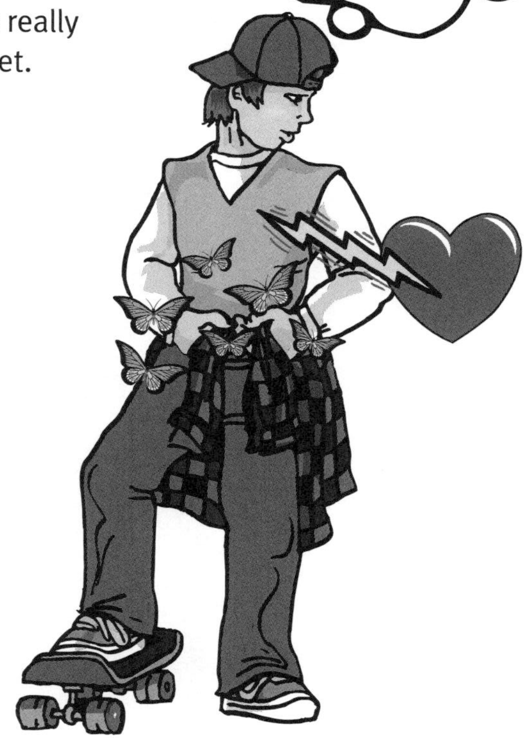

Help out Matthew

Write down what he could do to help his body's alarm chain reaction.
(Hint: Make sure to include calming activities and helpful thoughts.
You can use the **Strategies for Calming Down and Facing Fears** worksheet.)

1. ______________________________

____

2. ______________________________

____

3. ______________________________

____

4. ______________________________

____

5. ______________________________

____

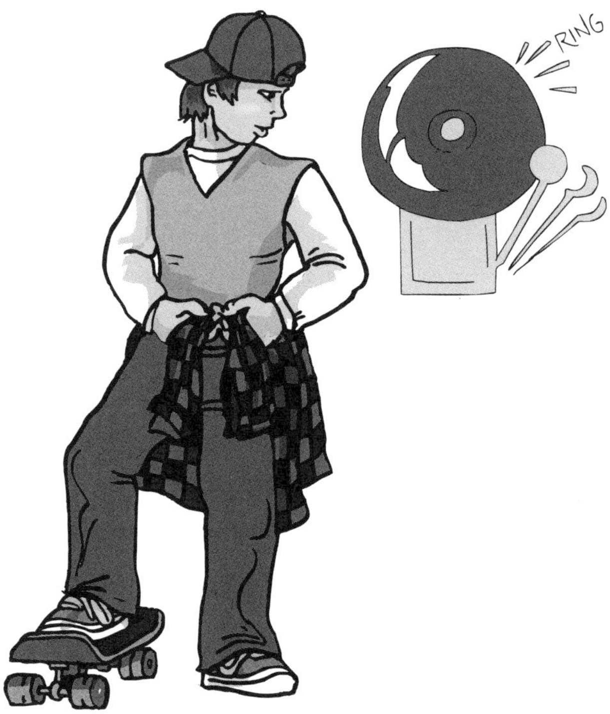

My Alarm Chain Reaction

Worry: ______________________________

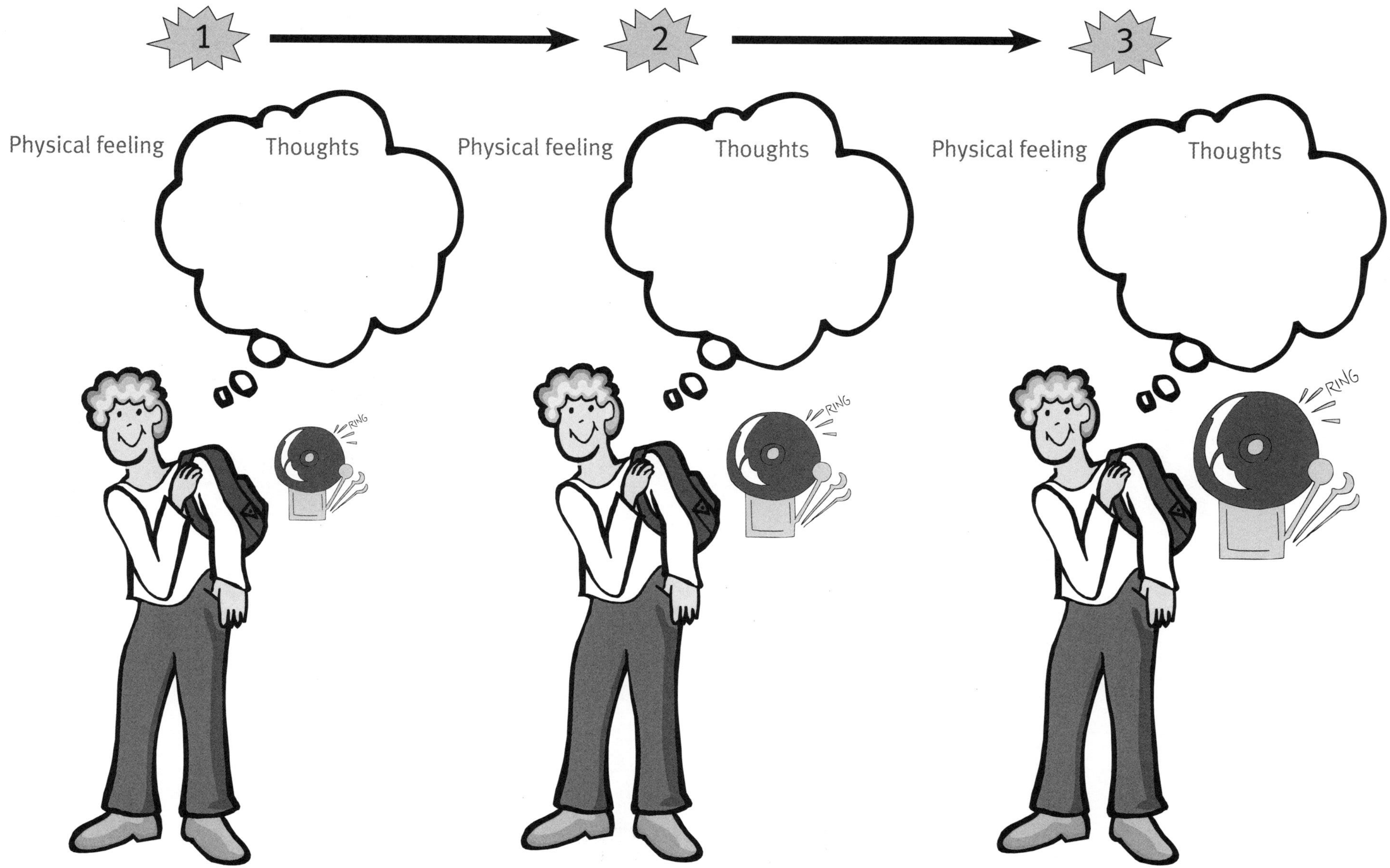

What Can I Do to Help Myself?

What could you do differently to help your body's alarm chain reaction?
(Hint: Make sure to include calming activities and helpful thoughts.
You can use the **Strategies for Calming Down and Facing Fears** worksheet.)

1. ____

____

2. ____

____

3. ____

____

4. ____

____

5. ____

____

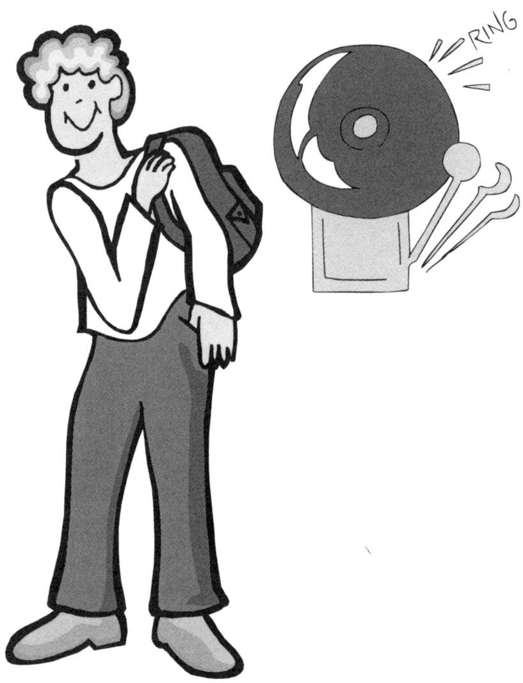

Strategies for Calming Down and Facing Fears

Suggestions for helpful thoughts:

- This is just a "false alarm."
- I can face my fear; nothing bad will happen.
- The worry feelings will go away.
- Fight back with facts.
- I can handle this.
- This is no big deal.
- Everyone makes mistakes.
- It's my worry bug; I can squash it!

Suggestions for calming activities:

- Take deep breaths.
- Go for a walk.
- Go outside.
- Ride my bike.
- Play with my pet.
- Read a book or magazine.
- Play video games.
- Watch television or a movie.
- Play with Lego set.
- Talk to someone.
- Play a game.
- Listen to music.
- Think about my favorite interest or activity.

Facing Fear of Snakes at the Zoo

Matthew wants to go on a field trip with his class to the zoo, but he is scared of snakes. Help him face his fear of snakes by creating **Steps to Success** and writing them on the lines below.

(Begin with Step 1 and move to Step 6)

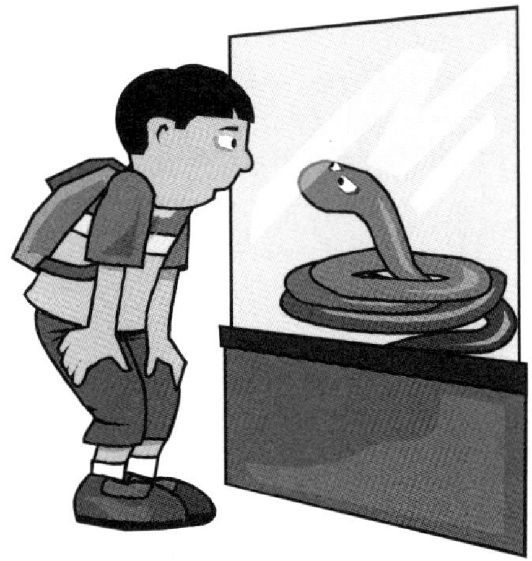

6. ______________________________

5. ______________________________

4. ______________________________

3. ______________________________

2. ______________________________

1. ______________________________

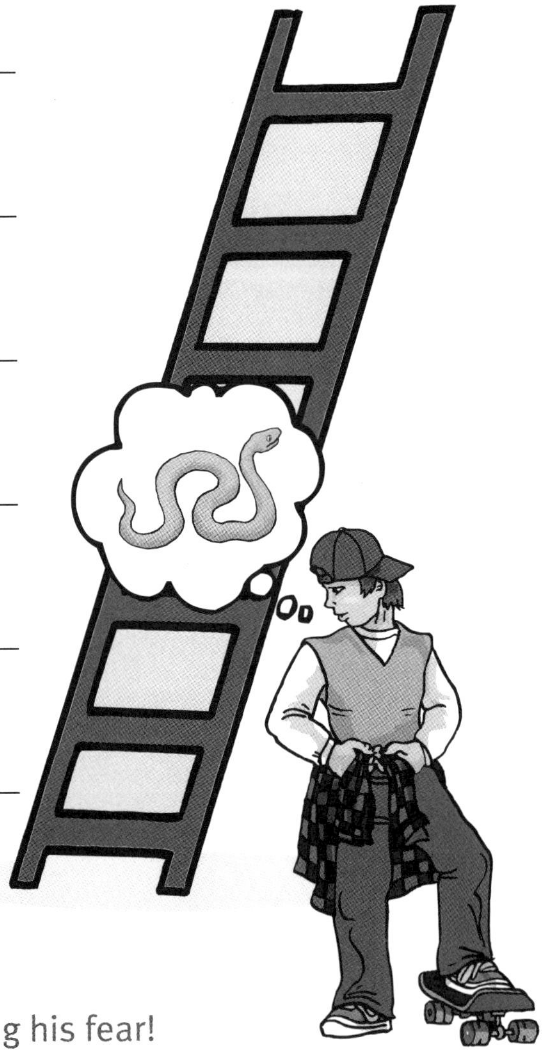

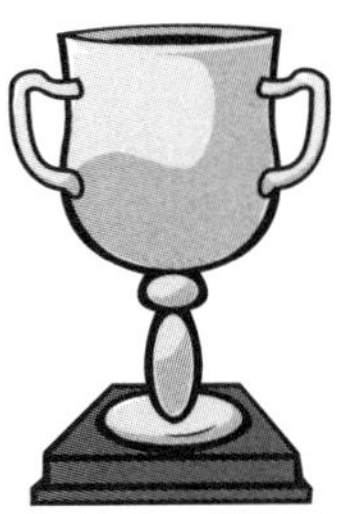

Matthew did an AWESOME job facing his fear!

REWARD!

Facing Fear of Talking in Class

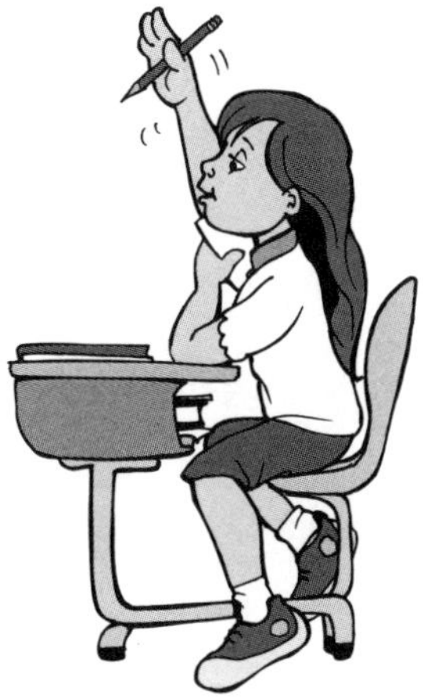

Susie likes science but is afraid to talk in class. Help her face her fear of talking in class by creating **Steps to Success** and writing them on the lines below.

(Begin with Step 1 and move to Step 6)

6. ______________________________

5. ______________________________

4. ______________________________

3. ______________________________

2. ______________________________

1. ______________________________

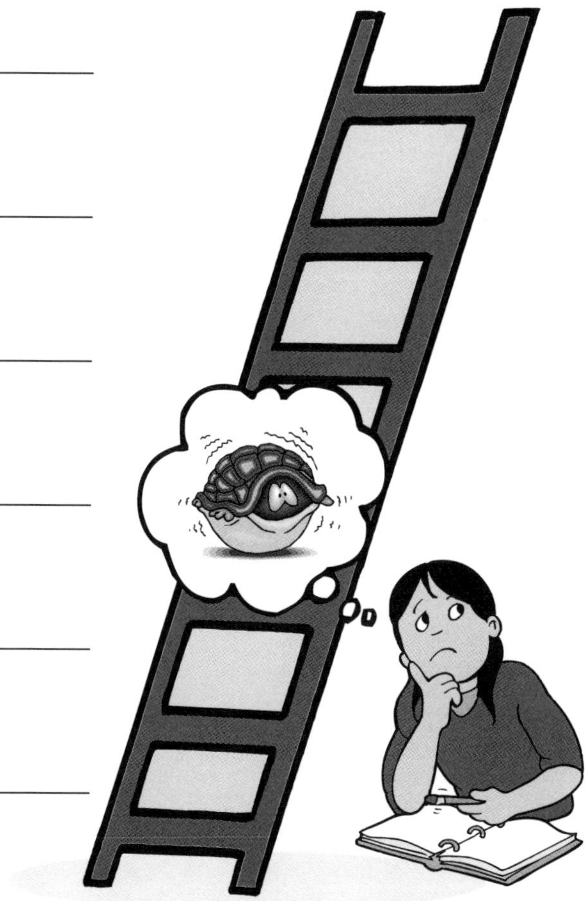

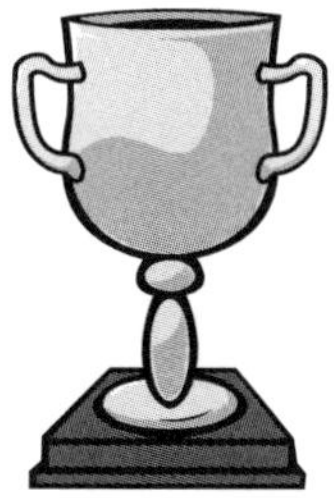

Susie did an AWESOME job facing her fear!

REWARD!

On the next page, together with your mom or dad, choose a goal to work on.

It may help to review your **Steps to Success: Finding My Target** and **Fear Tracker** worksheets to determine which fear to address first. Begin to write small steps that you can practice to help you face your fear and achieve your goal.

Next, talk with your mom or dad about what your reward will be when you reach the top of the ladder to success! What will you do to handle your worry when you are working on your goal and facing fears?

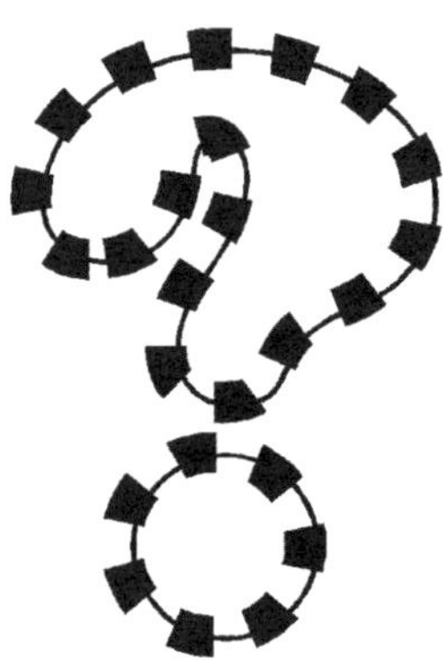

Steps to Success: Where Do We Begin?

What I'm working on (target goal): ____________________

What I'm working for (bigger reward!): ____________________

My reward for every exposure practice will be (small reward): ____________________

I will practice facing my fears (how often?): ____________________

(Begin with Step 1 and move to Step 6)

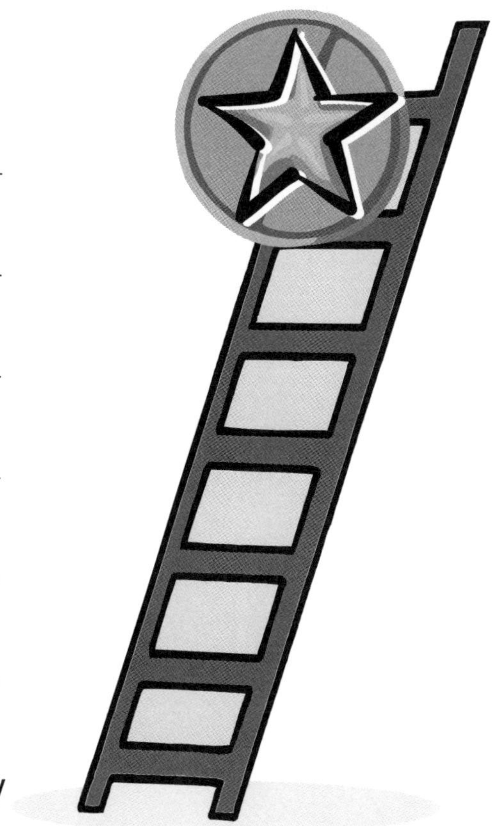

6. ____________________

5. ____________________

4. ____________________

3. ____________________

2. ____________________

1. ____________________

Strategies for Success! What I can do to handle my worry and/or fear at home (e.g., deep breathing):

1. ____________________

2. ____________________

3. ____________________

4. ____________________

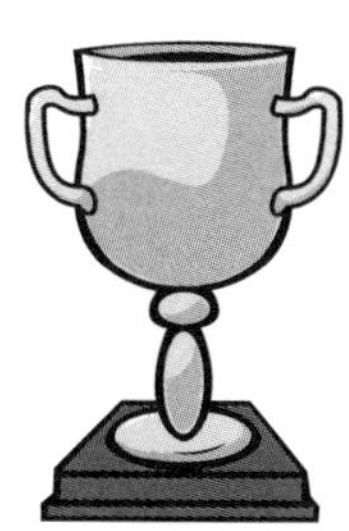

YOU DID IT!

Session 7

Introduction to Exposure

(Continued)

Facing Fears Rating Sheet

Name: ____________________

Session: ____________________

Date: ____________________

Fear: ____________________

Step to complete today in facing fears: ____________________

____

Reward for exposure practice: ____________________

	Child anxiety rating	Parent rates child anxiety
Before exposure		
During exposure		
Immediately after exposure		
5 minutes after exposure		

Facing Fears: How Did I Do?

1. How well did I face my fears? 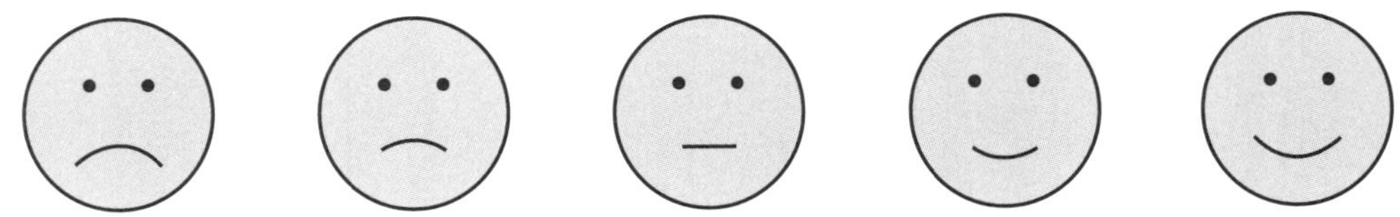

2. How well did I use my tools? 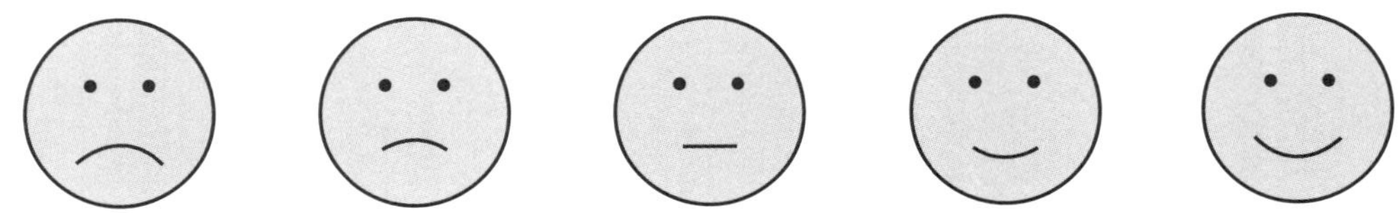

3. What will I do differently next time? ______________________________

____

____

____

Remember, look in your stress-o-meter to help you decide what to do next time!
Wow! Good job!

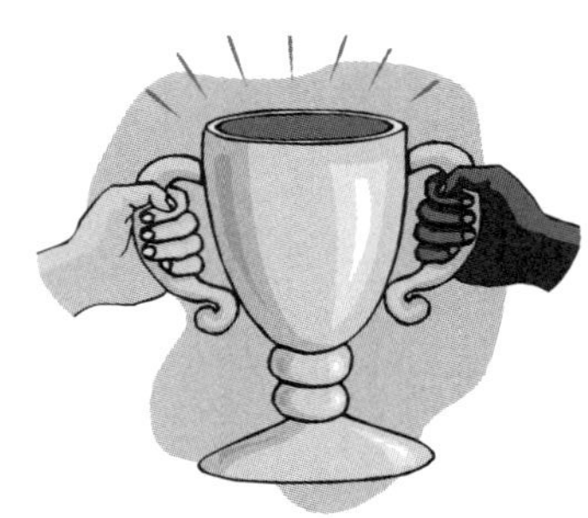

On the **Plan for My Movie** worksheet on the next page, you are going to choose the plot for your own movie!

Think about which of your worries you would like to target in your movie!

What will the steps to success be?
What will the plan be for calming down?
What will the reward be for facing your fear?
Where will your movie take place?
Who will the characters be?

Have fun planning your movie!

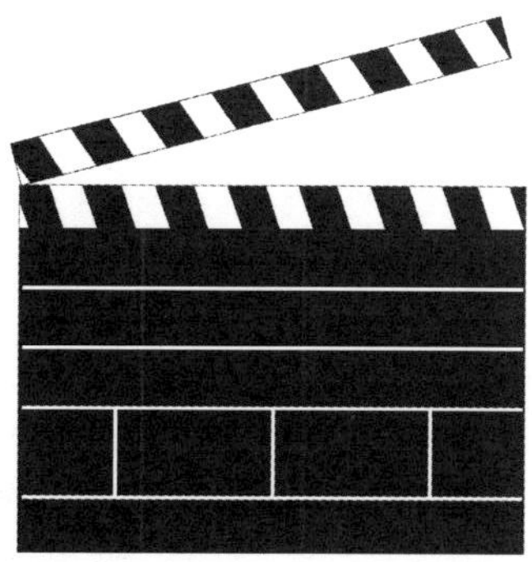

Plan for My Movie!

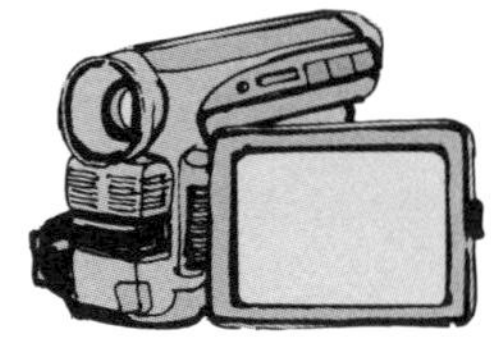

Specific worry or fear: ______________________________

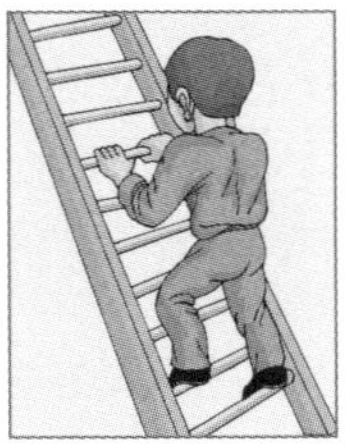

Steps to success
(facing fears a little at a time):

1. ______________________

2. ______________________

3. ______________________

4. ______________________

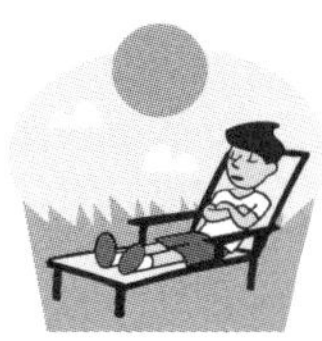

Strategies: (Hint: Make sure to include calming activities and helpful thoughts.)

____

____

____

____

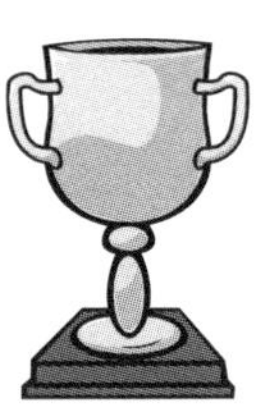

REWARDS! ______________________

____

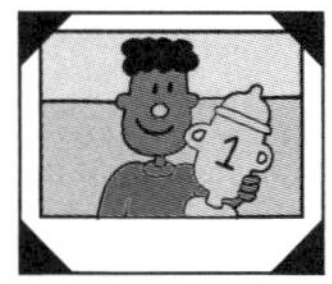

Self-praise: ______________________

____

____

Props: ______________________

____

____

Setting: ______________________

____

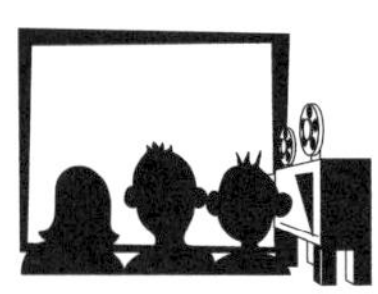

Roles:

1. Fear Facer: ______________________

2. Coach: ______________________

3. Narrator: ______________________

4. Other: ______________________

Sample Script:
Facing Your Fears: ______________

Narrator: Greetings. In our *Facing Your Fears* segment today, we are going to help you conquer your fear of ______________. We will introduce you to ______________, who is afraid of ______________. To help ______________ with his fear of ______________, his friend ______________ will coach him through the "steps to success." ______________ will start with Step 1— ______________________________
____.

Child #1: Ok, I'm ready to face my fear of ______________. I'll start by______________________
____.

Coach: Say, "I can do this—I want to beat this fear."

Child #1: I can do this. I want to beat this fear.

Coach: Where are you on your stress-o-meter?

Child #1: I'm starting to feel a little funny in my stomach; I think I'm at about a 6.

Coach: Try to get back down to a 4. Take a few deep breaths.

Child #1: (Takes a few breaths.)

Coach: Say, ______________(provides suggestions for handling anxiety, such as helpful thoughts, and/or suggestions for calming/relaxing activities) ____________________
____

Child #1: (Does suggestions) Now I think I am at about a 4.

Coach: Say, "I did it! Good for me, I finished the first step."

Child #1: I did it! Good for me, I finished the first step.

Narrator: (Child #1) ______________'s next step is to ______________________________
____.

Child #1: I am ready to do the second step. I am ready to ______________________________. I'm starting to feel a little worried.

Coach: Tell yourself, "Oh, it's just my worry bug again. I can fight this."

Child #1: Oh, it's just my worry bug again. I can fight this, but I feel like I am at a 7. Ahhh, I don't know what to do!

(continued)

(continued)

Sample Script:
Facing Your Fears: ________________

Coach: Take a few deep breaths.

Child #1: (Pauses and takes three deep breaths.)

Coach: You need to remember "helpful thoughts."

Child #1: I am strong. ______________________________
(Thinks helpful thoughts, such as "fight back with facts," or task-neutral thoughts).
I know the worry feelings will go away. Hey, it's working. I feel better.

Narrator: (Child #1) ______________'s next step is to ______________________________
______________________________.

Child #1: I am ready to ______________________________.
This is the hardest part, and I'm having trouble doing this! I feel like yelling.

Coach: Remember helpful thoughts. You can say, ______________________.
Tell yourself the worry feelings will go away.

Child #1: (Uses steps from plan.)

Child #1: I did it! I am proud of myself for not freaking out. I think I am at a 3.

Narrator: Now, (Child #1) ______________'s final step is to ______________.

Child #1: Now it's time for my final step. I am going to face my fear of ______________ and ______________. Oh no, my worry is going up to an 8 this time.

Coach: Say, "I can do this." You need to calm yourself down. Take three deep breaths.

Child #1: I can do this. (Takes 3 deep breaths.) This will be over in a few minutes.

Child #1: I did it. I faced my fear of ______________ and my worry passed. I did a good job!
I'm proud of myself. I think I'll reward myself with ______________________.

Coach: Great job! (High five.)

Narrator: Now, all of you have a plan for facing your fear of ______________________.
I'll see you next time on another episode of *Facing Your Fears!*

Session 8

Practicing Exposure and Making Movies

Facing Fears Rating Sheet

Name: ______________________________

Session: ______________________________

Date: ______________________________

Fear: ______________________________

Step to complete today in facing fears: ______________________________

____

Reward for exposure practice: ______________________________

	Child anxiety rating	Parent rates child anxiety
Before exposure		
During exposure		
Immediately after exposure		
5 minutes after exposure		

Facing Fears: How Did I Do?

1. How well did I face my fears?

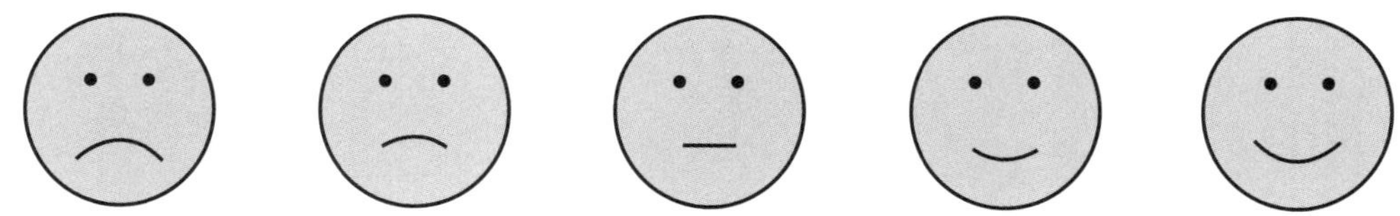

2. How well did I use my tools?

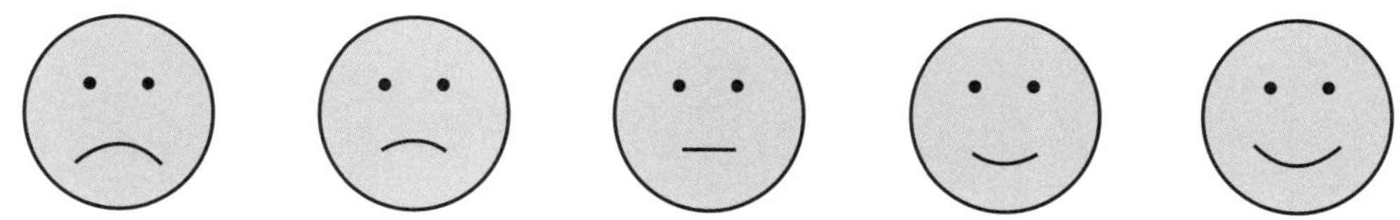

3. What will I do differently next time? ______________________

____

____

____

Remember, look in your stress-o-meter to help you decide what to do next time!
Wow! Good job!

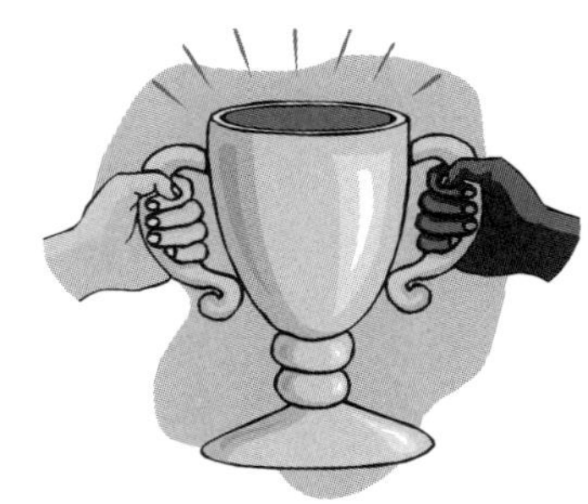

Things to Think About While Filming Our Movies!

Goals

How are you doing on your ***goals*** at home?
Keep at it! You're doing great!

Relax and have fun

Are you planning fun activities and time to relax? Try to plan some fun things to do during the week and calming or relaxing activities.

Are you ready to ***film*** your movie?
Do you need props? What else do you need?

Filming

Have fun with your movies, and good luck with your goals at home!

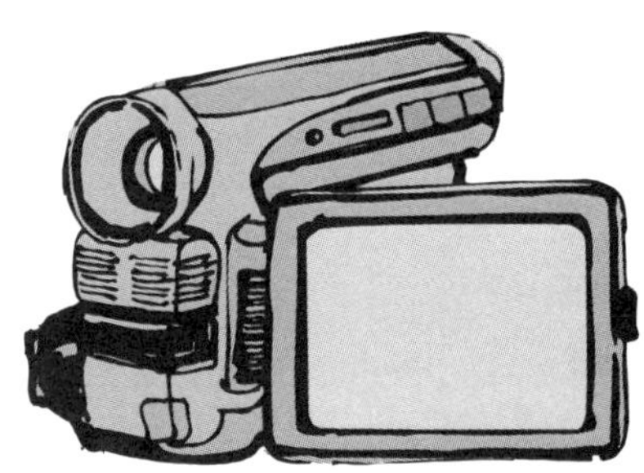

Session
9

Facing Fears and Making Movies

Facing Fears Rating Sheet

Name: ____

Session: ____

Date: ____

Fear: ____

Step to complete today in facing fears: ______________________________

____

Reward for exposure practice: ______________________________

	Child anxiety rating	Parent rates child anxiety
Before exposure		
During exposure		
Immediately after exposure		
5 minutes after exposure		

Facing Fears: How Did I Do?

1. How well did I face my fears?

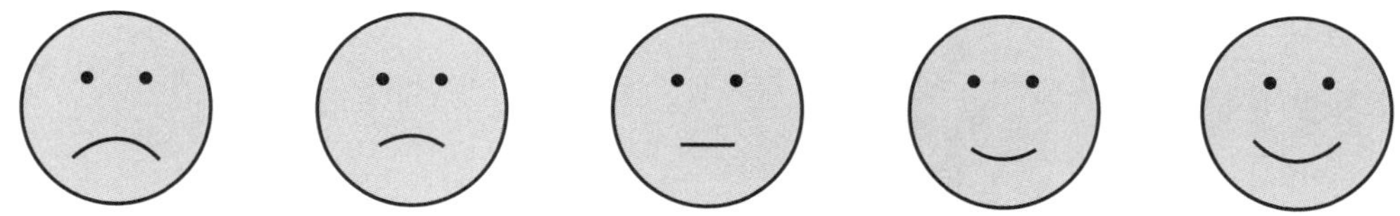

2. How well did I use my tools?

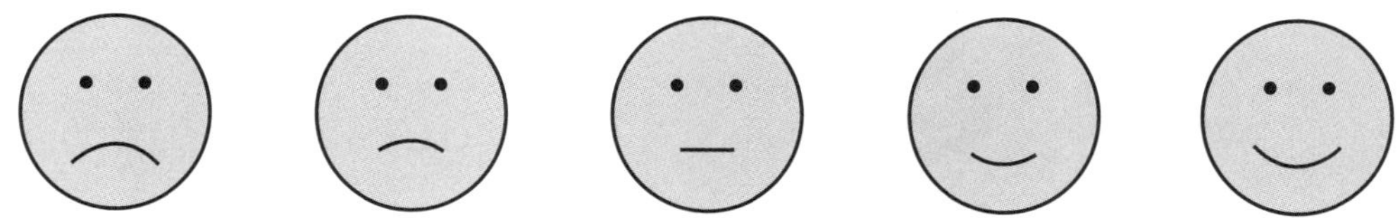

3. What will I do differently next time? ____________________

____

____

____

Remember, look in your stress-o-meter to help you decide what to do next time!
Wow! Good job!

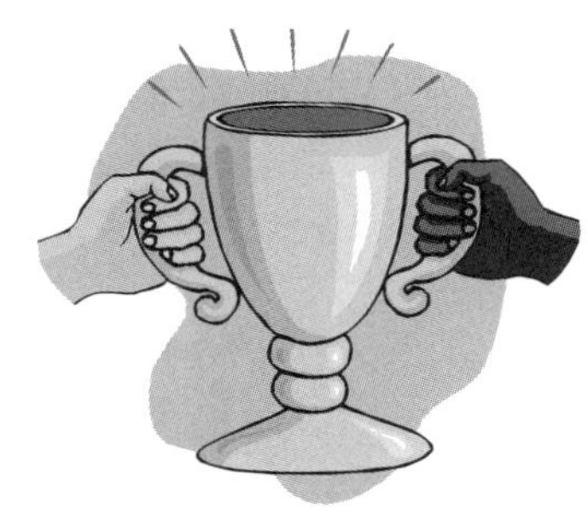

Session 10

Facing Fears and Making Movies

Facing Fears Rating Sheet

Name: ______________________________

Session: ______________________________

Date: ______________________________

Fear: ______________________________

Step to complete today in facing fears: ______________________________

____

Reward for exposure practice: ______________________________

	Child anxiety rating	Parent rates child anxiety
Before exposure		
During exposure		
Immediately after exposure		
5 minutes after exposure		

Facing Fears: How Did I Do?

1. How well did I face my fears? 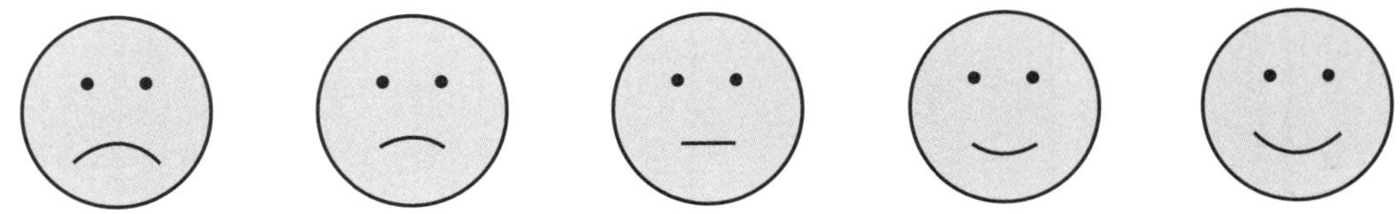

2. How well did I use my tools? 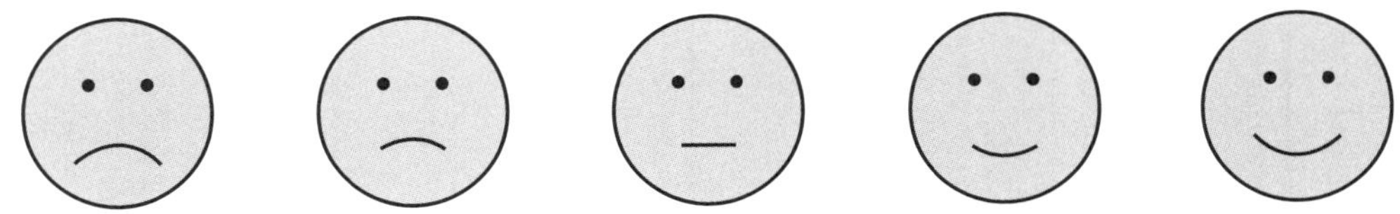

3. What will I do differently next time? ______________________________

____

____

____

Remember, look in your stress-o-meter to help you decide what to do next time!
Wow! Good job!

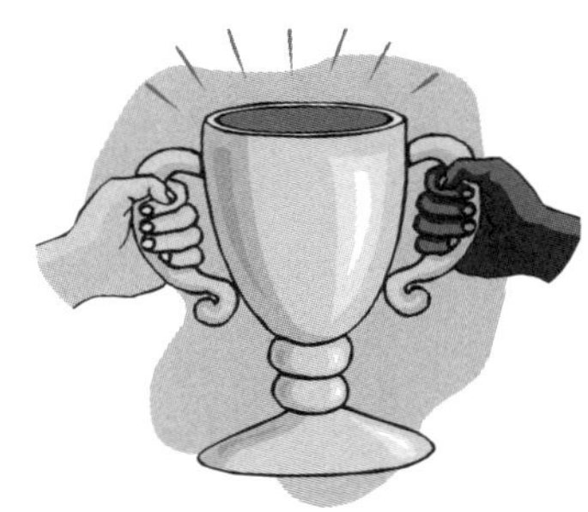

Session 11

Facing Fears and Making Movies

Facing Fears Rating Sheet

Name: ____________________

Session: ____________________

Date: ____________________

Fear: ____________________

Step to complete today in facing fears: ____________________

____

Reward for exposure practice: ____________________

	Child anxiety rating	Parent rates child anxiety
Before exposure		
During exposure		
Immediately after exposure		
5 minutes after exposure		

Facing Fears: How Did I Do?

1. How well did I face my fears? 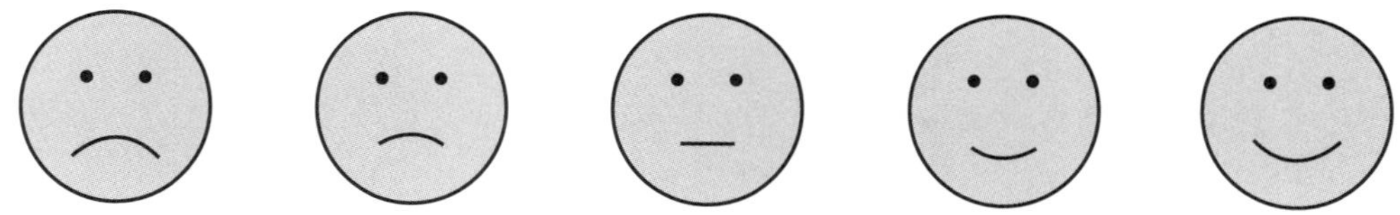

2. How well did I use my tools? 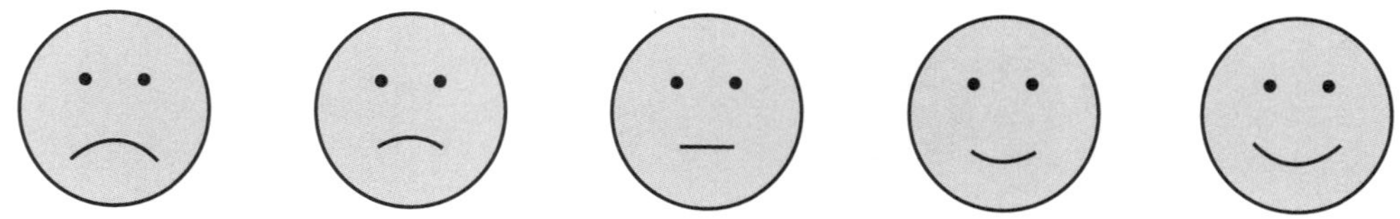

3. What will I do differently next time? ______

______

______

______

Remember, look in your stress-o-meter to help you decide what to do next time!
Wow! Good job!

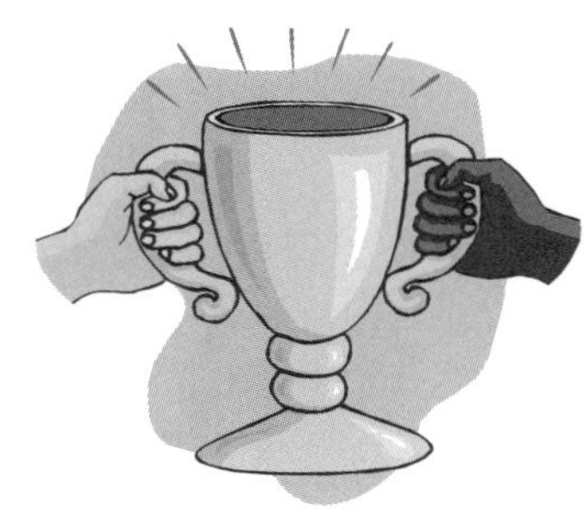

Session 12

Facing Fears and Making Movies

Facing Fears Rating Sheet

Name: ______________________________

Session: ______________________________

Date: ______________________________

Fear: ______________________________

Step to complete today in facing fears: ______________________________

____

Reward for exposure practice: ______________________________

	Child anxiety rating	Parent rates child anxiety
Before exposure		
During exposure		
Immediately after exposure		
5 minutes after exposure		

Facing Fears: How Did I Do?

1. How well did I face my fears? 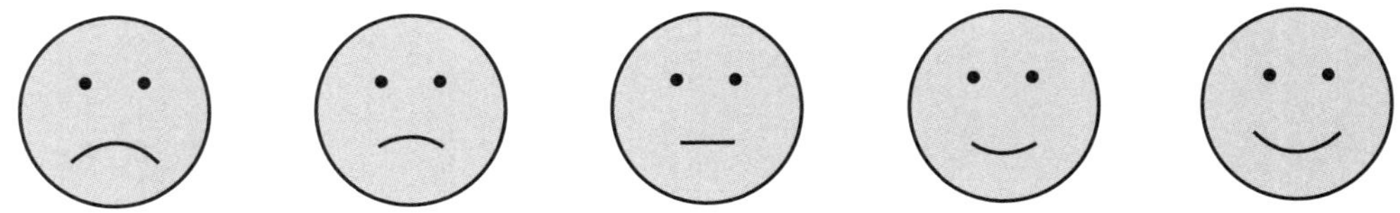

2. How well did I use my tools? 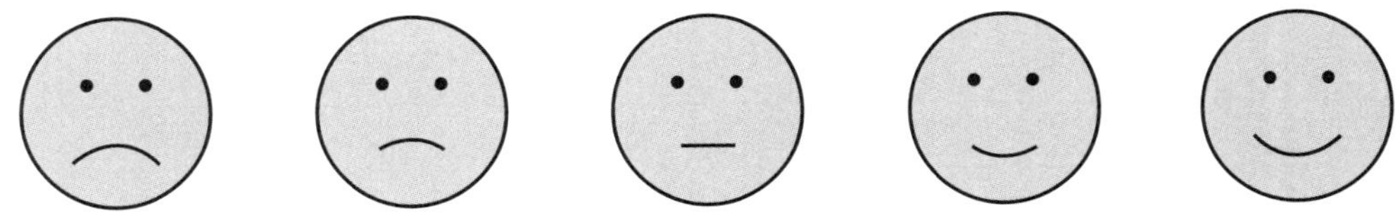

3. What will I do differently next time? ______________________________

____

____

____

Remember, look in your stress-o-meter to help you decide what to do next time!
Wow! Good job!

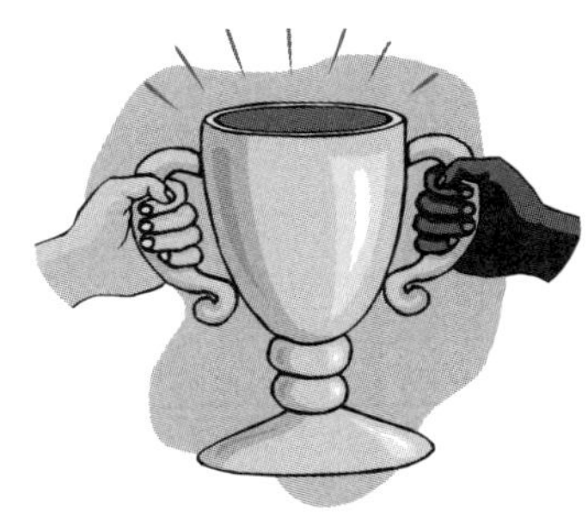

Session 13

Facing Fears and Making Movies

Facing Fears Rating Sheet

Name: ______________________________

Session: ______________________________

Date: ______________________________

Fear: ______________________________

Step to complete today in facing fears: ______________________________

____

Reward for exposure practice: ______________________________

	Child anxiety rating	Parent rates child anxiety
Before exposure		
During exposure		
Immediately after exposure		
5 minutes after exposure		

Facing Fears: How Did I Do?

1. How well did I face my fears?

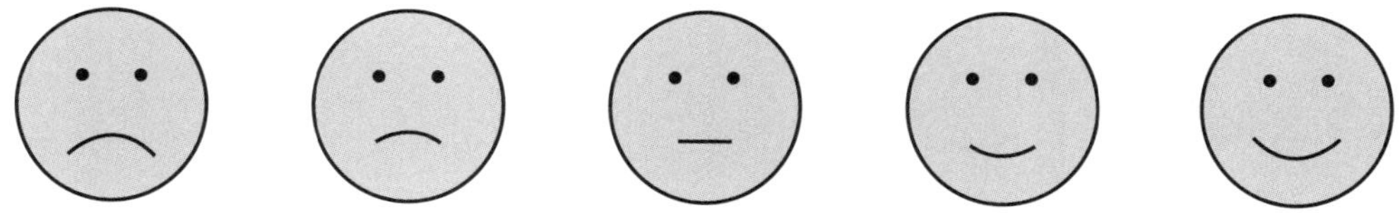

2. How well did I use my tools?

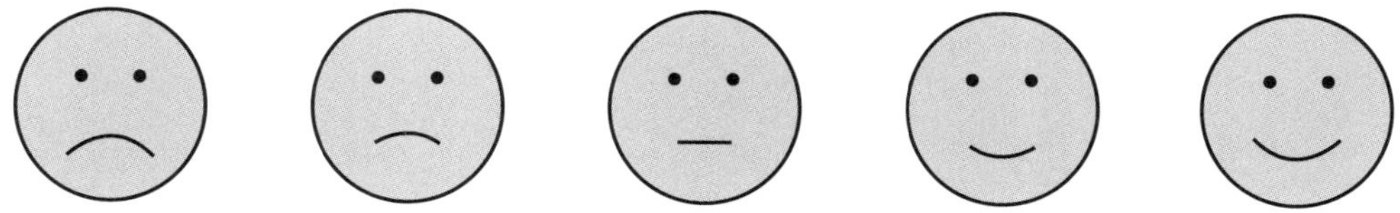

3. What will I do differently next time?

Remember, look in your stress-o-meter to help you decide what to do next time!
Wow! Good job!

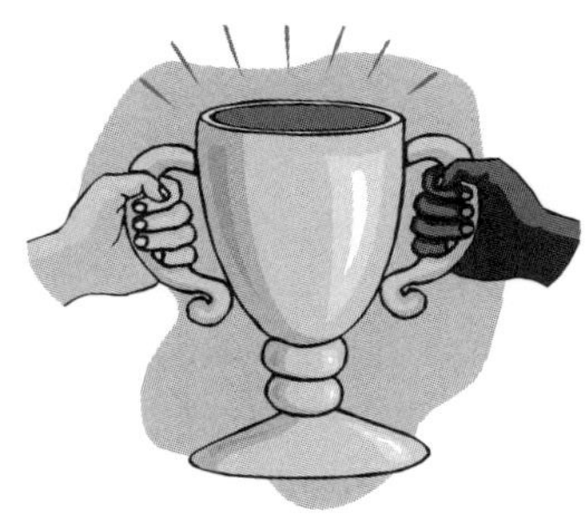

Session 14

Graduation

How Much Time Do You Spend Worrying Now?

Write down your worries here!

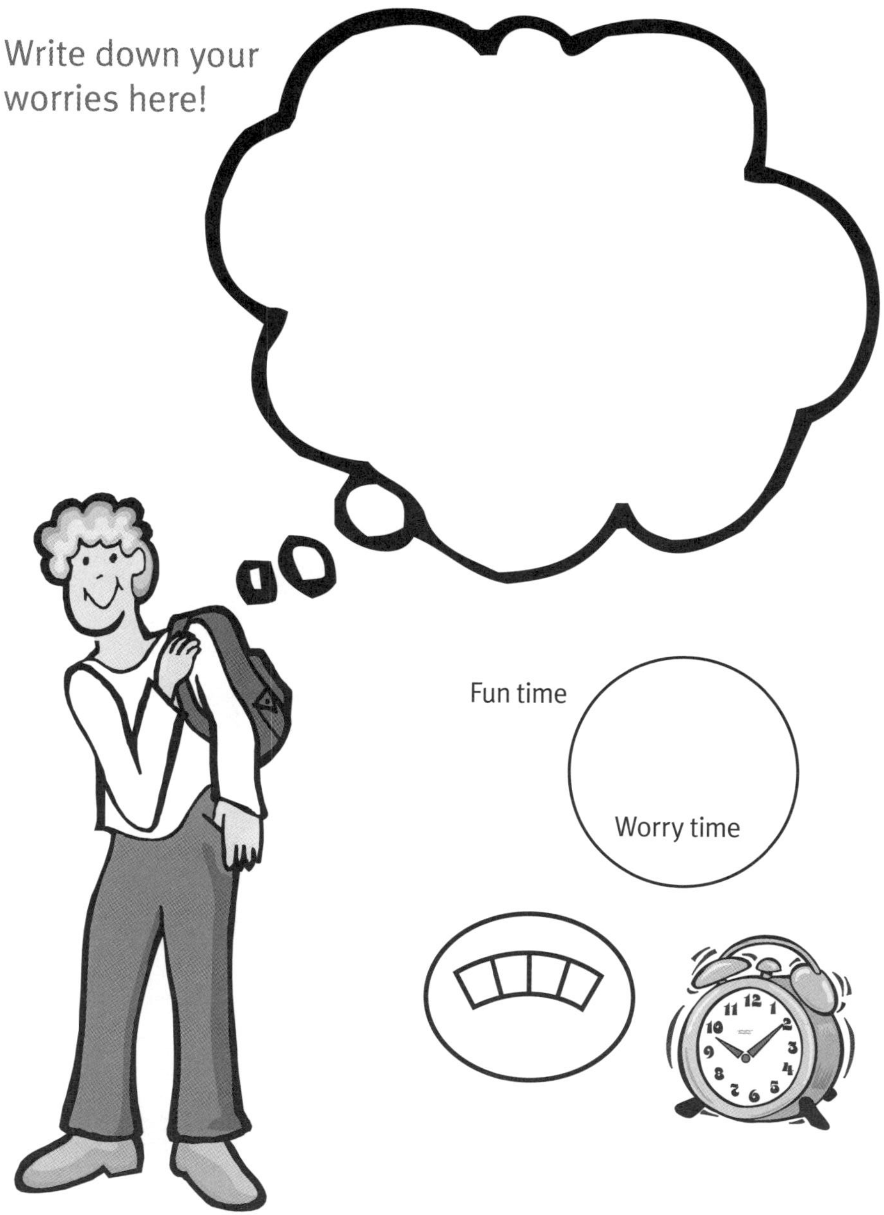

Time I spend worrying

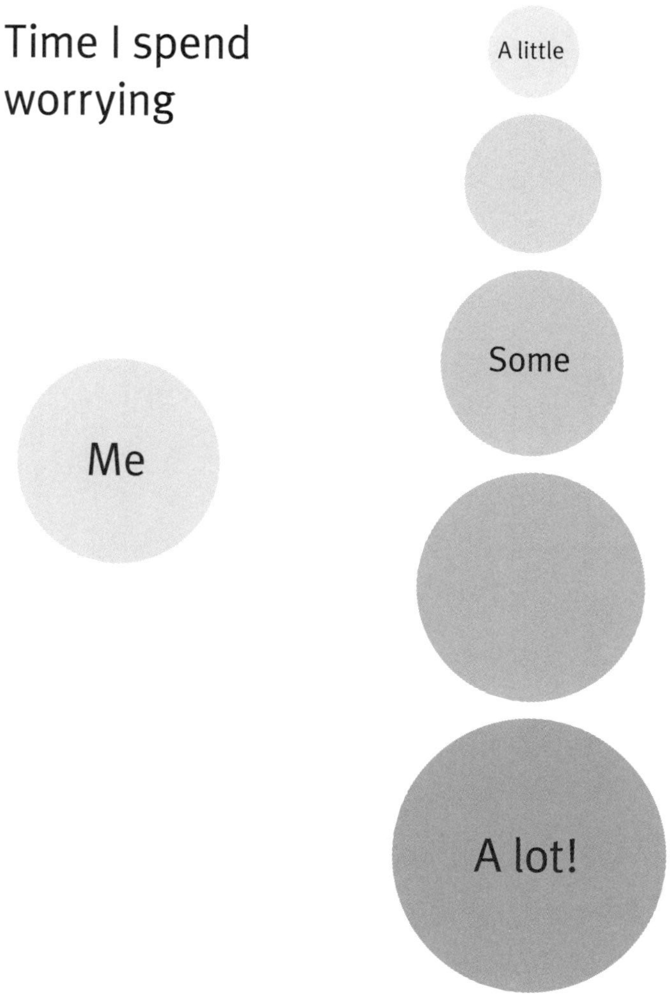

My Favorite Tools

Calming and/or relaxing activities

____

____

____

____

Helpful thoughts

____

____

____

____

I faced fears by . . .

____

____

____

____

____

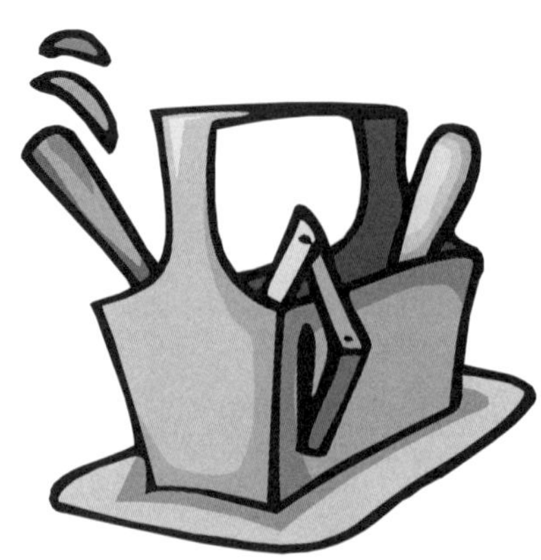

Lessons I Learned in Group

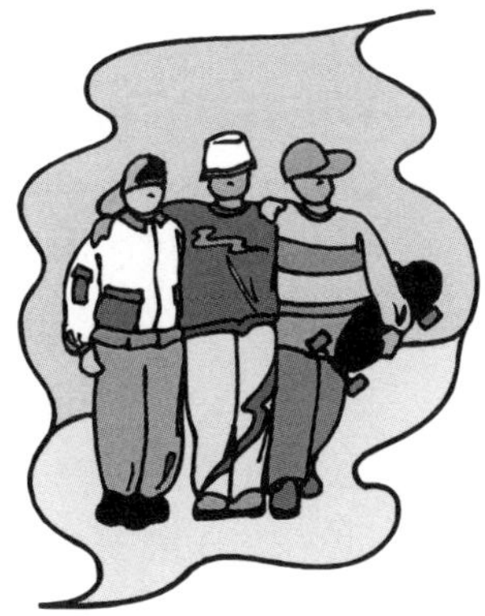

- We all use different words for worry—*scared, anxious, nervous,* and *freaked out* are some of them.
- When we worry too much, it can make it hard for us to have fun, do well in school, or get along with our family or friends.

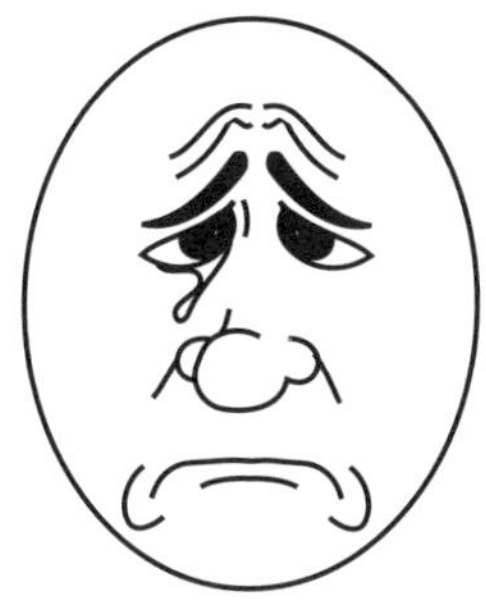

- Different things make each of us worry or feel anxious. It may be a fear of the dark, of going outside, of staying home alone, or of talking to people.
- We can show worry or anxiety in lots of different ways, such as getting really quiet, leaving the room, crying, getting silly, or even having our bodies shake.

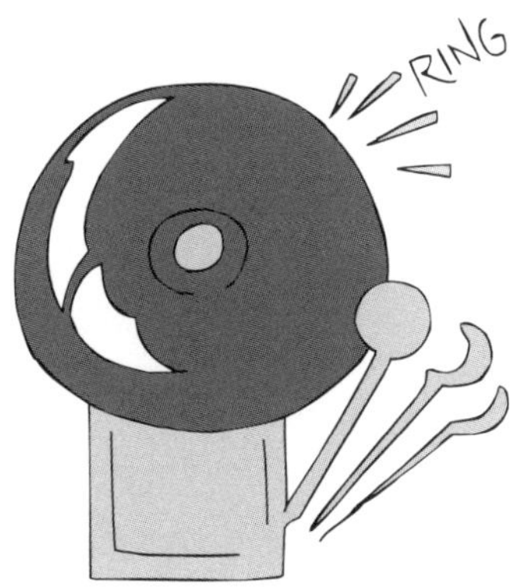

- Sometimes our worry is a "false alarm"—our bodies may feel upset, then our minds get really active and we start thinking all sorts of thoughts that make us worry more.
- It helps to know the kinds of situations that make us worry so we can get ready to fight it!

(continued)

(continued)

Lessons I Learned in Group

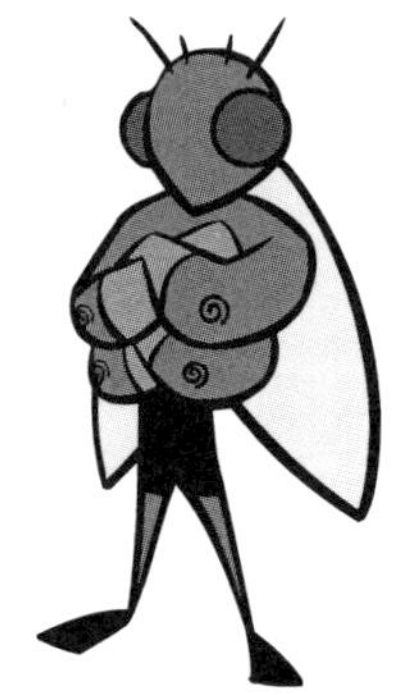

- We can do *lots* of things to get rid of worry. We can do relaxing and calming things like taking deep breaths, telling a joke, or going for a walk. We also can remember that helpful thoughts can make our bodies calm down. We can fight back with facts or tell ourselves that the worry feelings will go away. We can watch our favorite television shows, play video games, listen to music, ride bikes, read a book, or talk on the phone while we wait for our worry to go away.

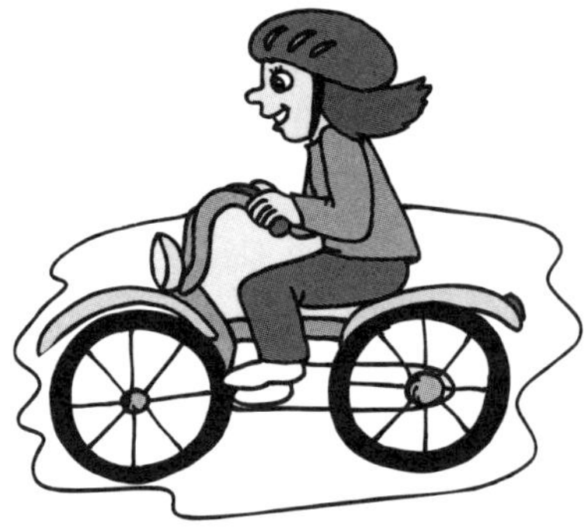

- We are all very strong and tough. We can beat worry!

- Most important, we learned that the best way to get rid of worry is to face fears!

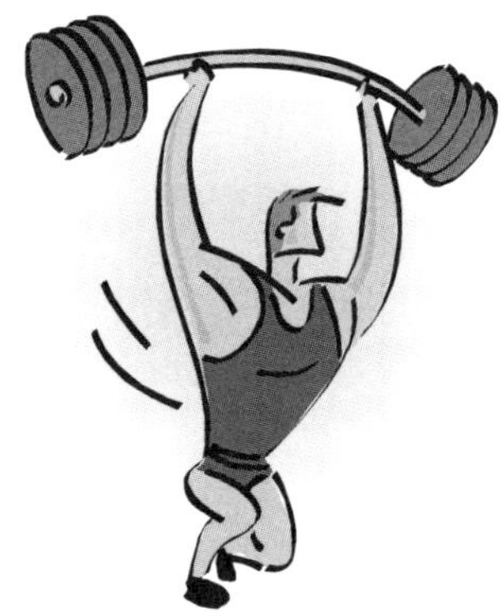

Favorite things I'll remember about my friends:

____

____

____

____

We learned a whole lot of different things in group!

Booster Session

You have worked hard to face your fears, but you may still have worries that get in your way of having fun or getting things done. Review the list on the next page and answer the following questions:

Which of these items do you worry about sometimes?
Which do you worry about a lot?
Which items do you never worry about?

After you read the list, decide with your mom or dad which kinds of things you continue to worry about. Transfer them to the **Steps to Success: Finding My Target** worksheet. If you do not have any big worries now, then you can leave this worksheet blank.

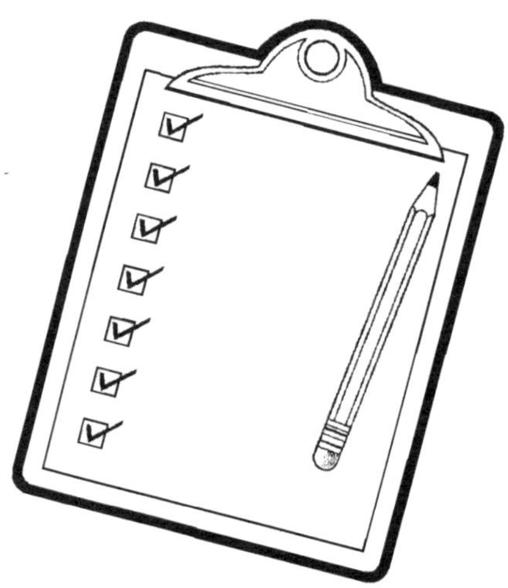

My Checklist of Fears, Worries, and Irritations

I'm afraid of, worried about, or irritated about . . .

	No	Sometimes	A lot	Stress-o-meter rating (1–8)
Being late				
Being home alone				
Making mistakes				
The dark				
Letting go of past events				
Dogs and/or cats				
Storms and/or tornados				
Bugs, spiders, and/or bees				
Getting a disease				
Being teased				
Germs				
Trying new foods				
Being away from family				
Using public bathrooms				
Talking to new people				
Talking in school				
Getting to sleep				
Scary movies				
Changes				
Asking for help				
Parents going out				
Getting lost				
Dying				
Starting homework				
World events				
Going to someone's house				
Loud noises				
Heights				
Starting a conversation				
Being in a room by myself				
Performing in front of others				
Other:				

Steps to Success: Finding My Target

____
Biggest worry

____
Pretty big worry

____
Medium worry

____
Bit of a worry

____
Not much of a worry

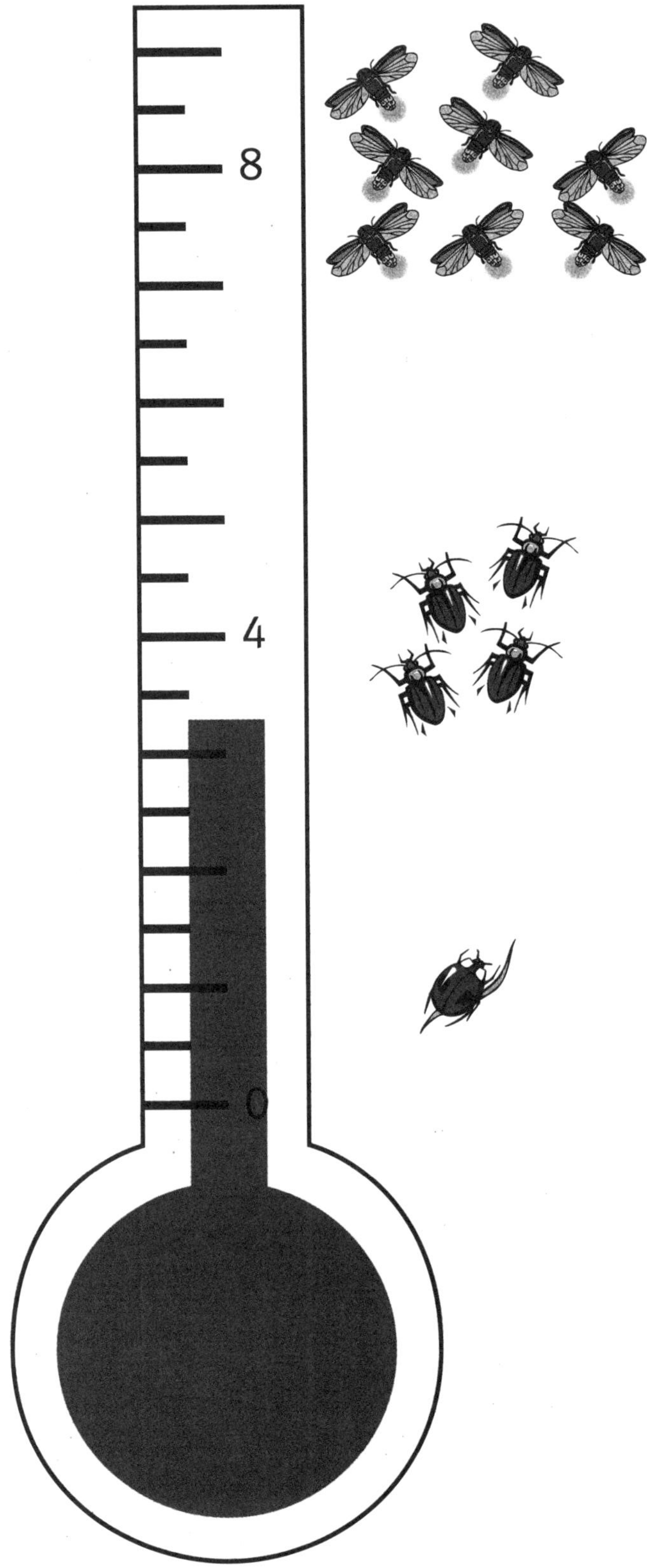

In group, you learned a lot of different strategies for facing fears or worry. Some of these strategies may work better than others. On the next page, write down your favorite tools for facing fears and handling worry. Then, look at the **Stressed to Calm** worksheet and think of how the boy can solve a problem using helpful thoughts, calming and/or relaxing activities, and facing fears strategies to calm himself.

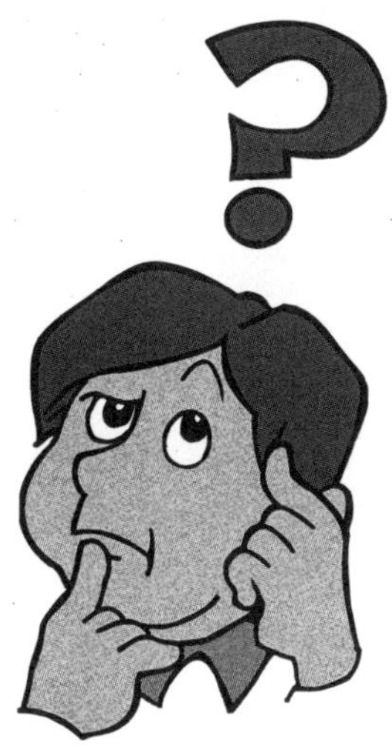

My Favorite Tools

Calming and/or relaxing activities

____

____

____

____

Helpful thoughts

____

____

____

____

I faced fears by . . .

____

____

____

____

____

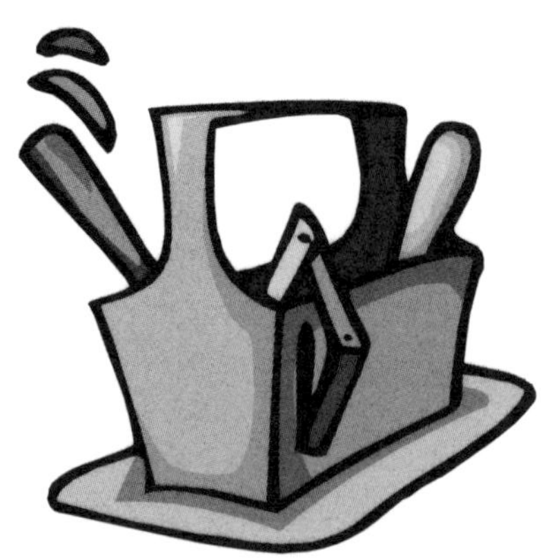

Stressed to Calm

Problem: ____

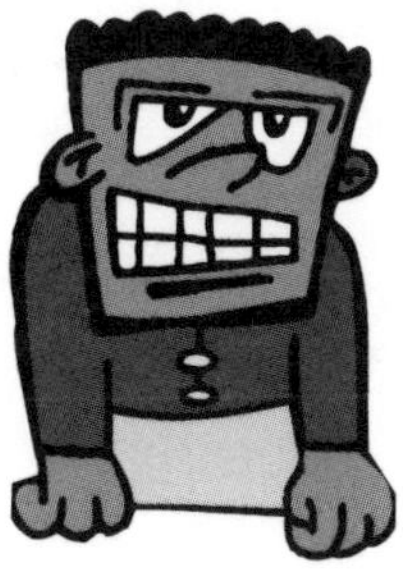

I think ______________

I feel ______________

Helpful thoughts

____

____

____

____

Calming and/or relaxing activities

____

____

____

____

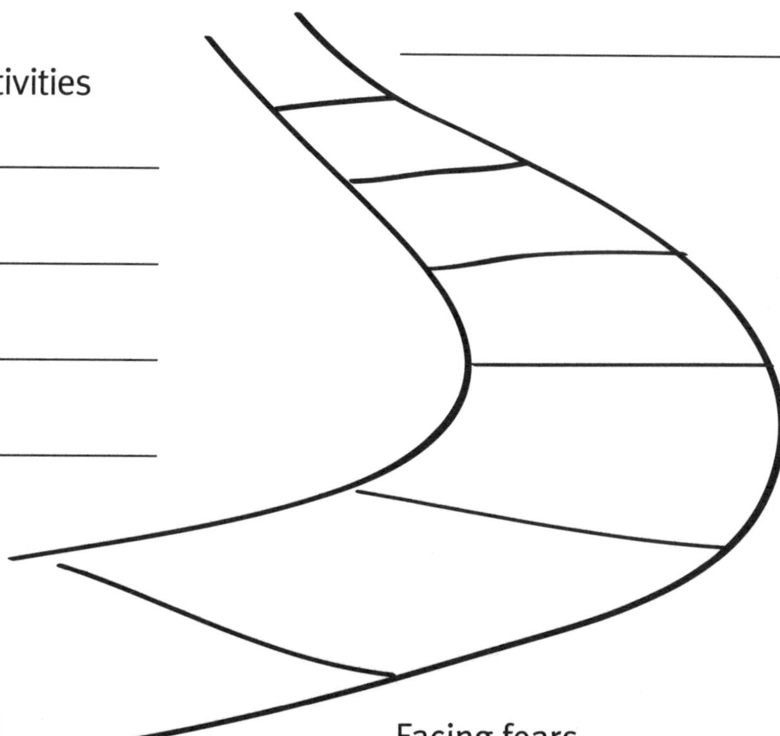

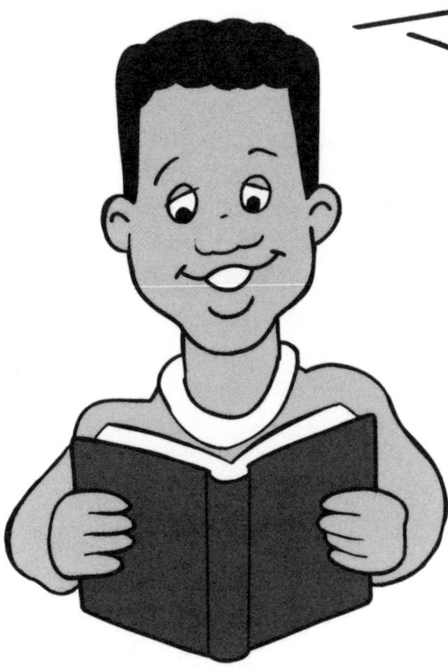

Facing fears

____

____

____

____

This workbook is part of *Facing Your Fears*, an innovative, family-focused group therapy program that helps children with high-functioning autism and Asperger syndrome conquer their anxiety—and participate more fully in home, school, and community life. The complete *Facing Your Fears* set (Facilitator's Manual, Parent Workbook, and Child Workbook—extra workbook packs sold separately) allows for the administration of 15 complete sessions for children 8–14 and their parents. See **www.brookespublishing.com** to learn more about *Facing Your Fears* and order the components.

ISBN-13: 978-1-59857-177-6
ISBN-10: 1-59857-177-X
Reorder in packs of 4 using 71806

·PAUL·H·
BROOKES
PUBLISHING CO®
www.brookespublishing.com

Welcome to Group

Words We Use for Worry

Words for Worry Word Search

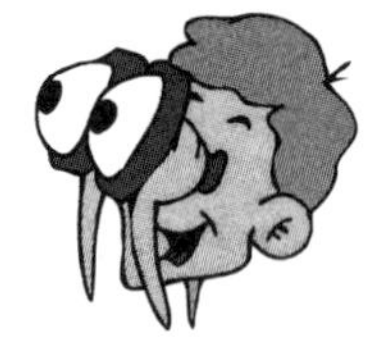

Everyone talks about worry in different ways.
Find the 12 words below that describe how people feel
when they are worried.

D	O	V	E	R	W	H	E	L	M	E	D	E	F	T
F	E	A	M	G	R	D	L	P	S	C	I	T	R	W
E	R	I	T	U	P	S	E	T	B	H	Z	J	I	O
A	T	C	E	Z	H	C	G	M	W	E	H	M	G	T
R	S	O	T	S	I	N	E	R	V	O	U	S	H	O
F	C	M	D	B	K	C	P	B	E	R	E	A	T	F
U	A	F	E	V	A	F	R	A	I	D	L	G	E	J
L	R	Q	H	L	R	N	I	P	G	V	Q	R	N	A
C	E	M	W	K	T	F	X	K	W	P	Z	A	E	G
B	D	H	O	F	S	D	B	I	T	S	Z	T	D	I
L	B	Y	R	A	G	T	O	V	O	E	F	L	Y	T
R	K	E	R	B	H	Z	M	W	R	U	A	M	I	A
A	G	F	Y	Y	E	C	S	K	N	L	S	J	W	T
L	M	R	G	J	K	W	J	E	T	R	Q	K	C	E
F	R	E	A	K	E	D	O	U	T	O	U	E	T	D

WORRY	SCARED	UPSET	FREAKED OUT
AFRAID	FRIGHTENED	ANXIOUS	MELTDOWN
NERVOUS	FEARFUL	AGITATED	OVERWHELMED

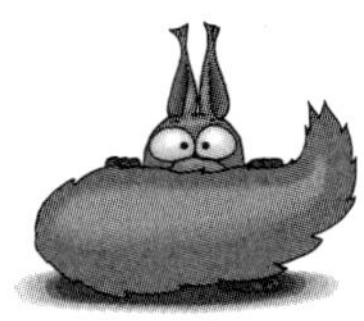

Did you find all the words?
What words do you use to describe how you feel sometimes?

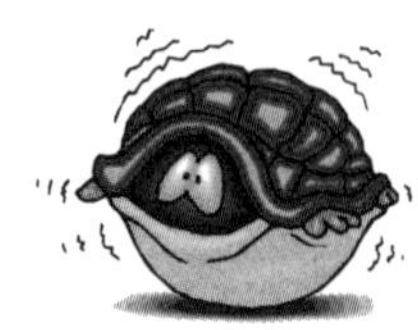

Time Michael Spends Worrying

Michael worries about a lot of different things. He spends a lot of his time during the day worrying!

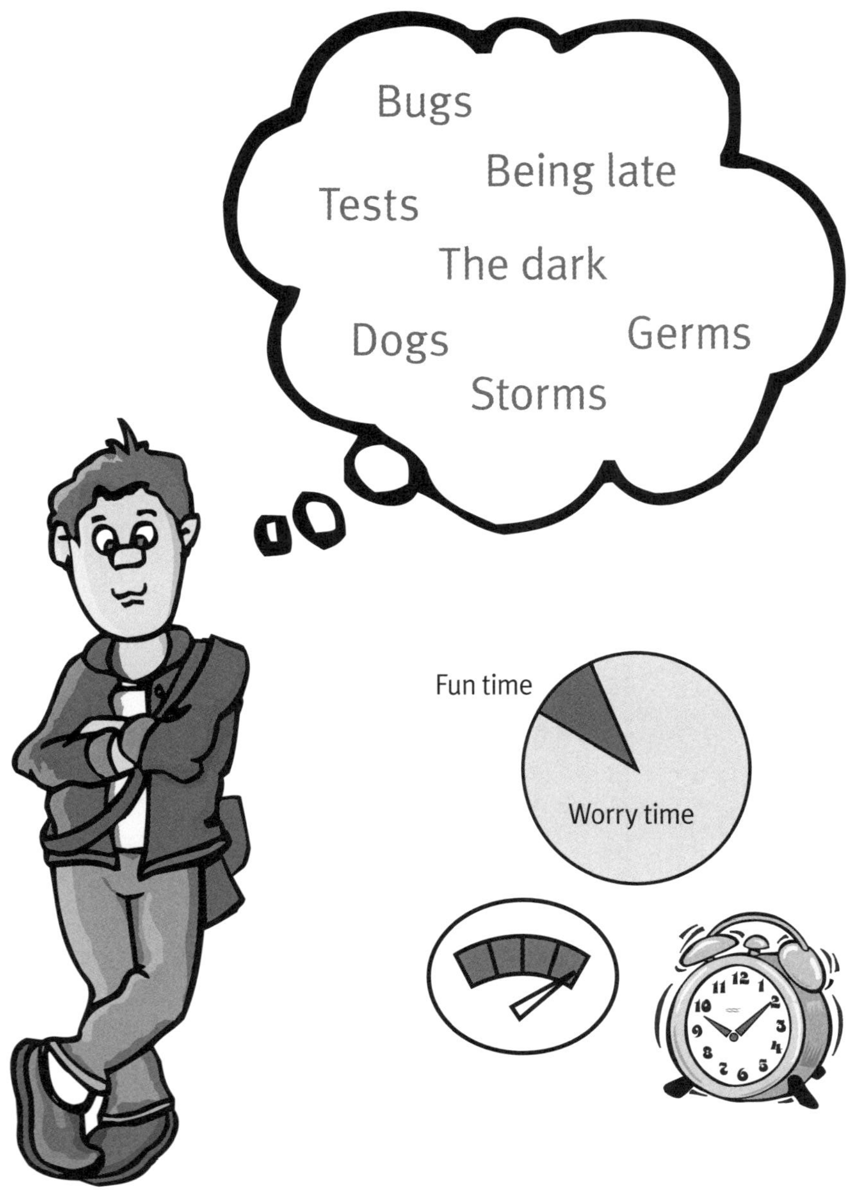

Time Michael spends worrying

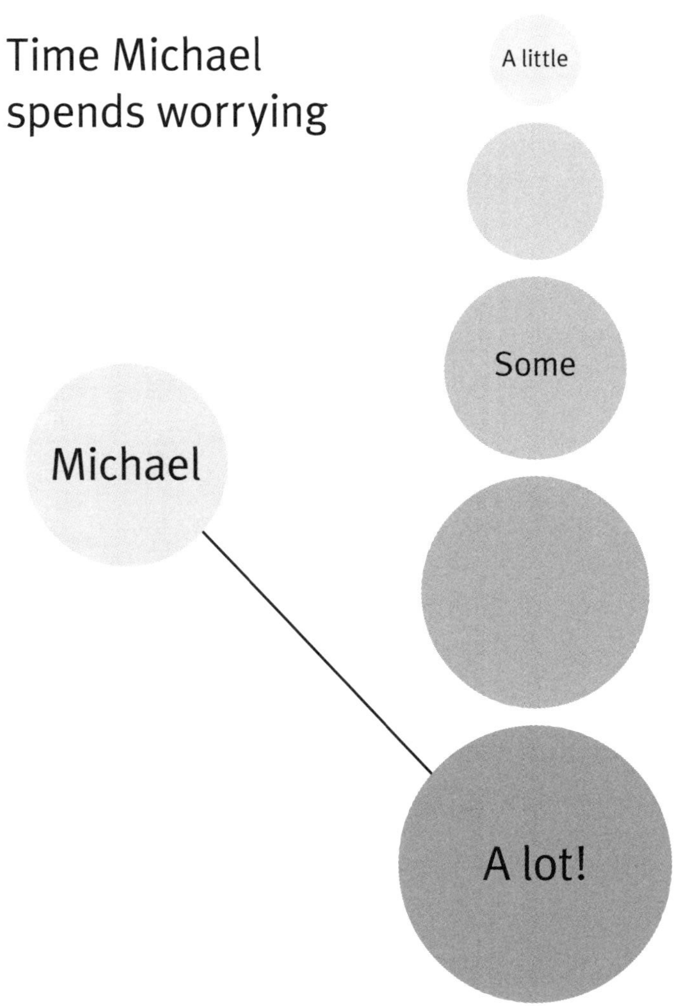

Michael has no time to do anything fun.
He spends almost all of his time worrying!

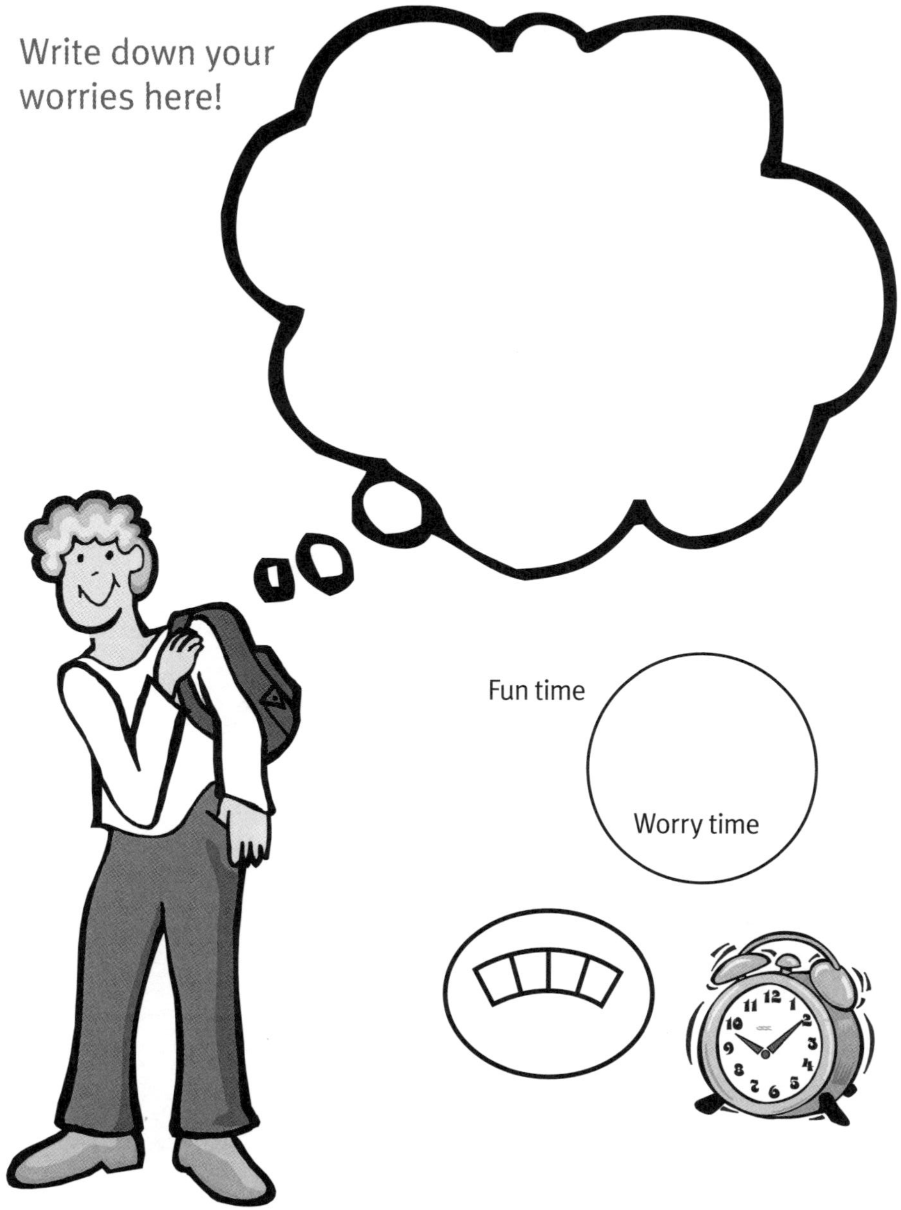

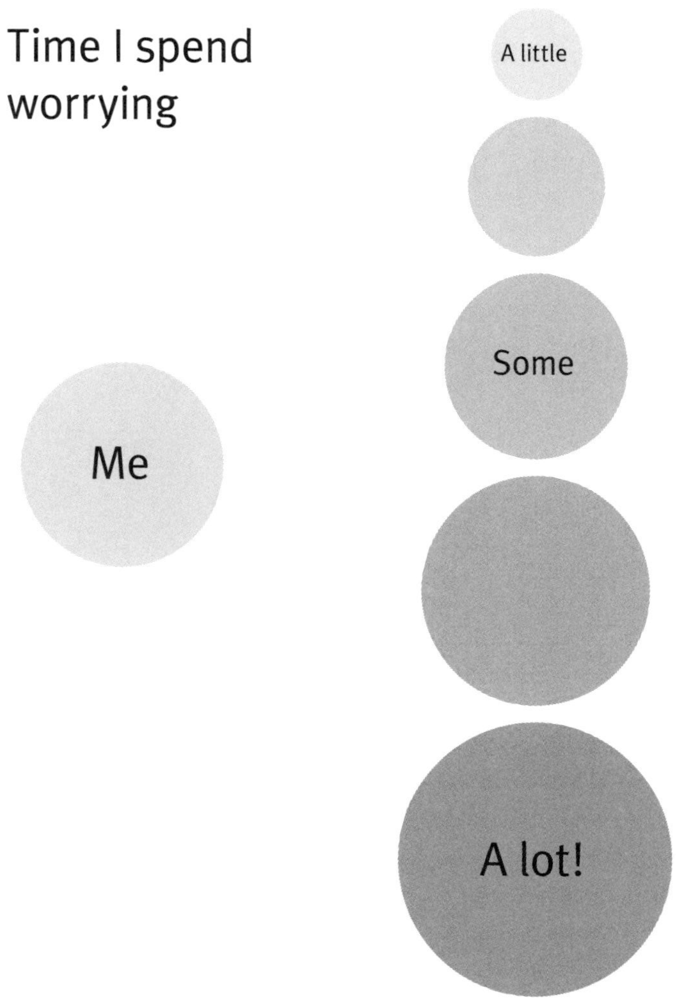

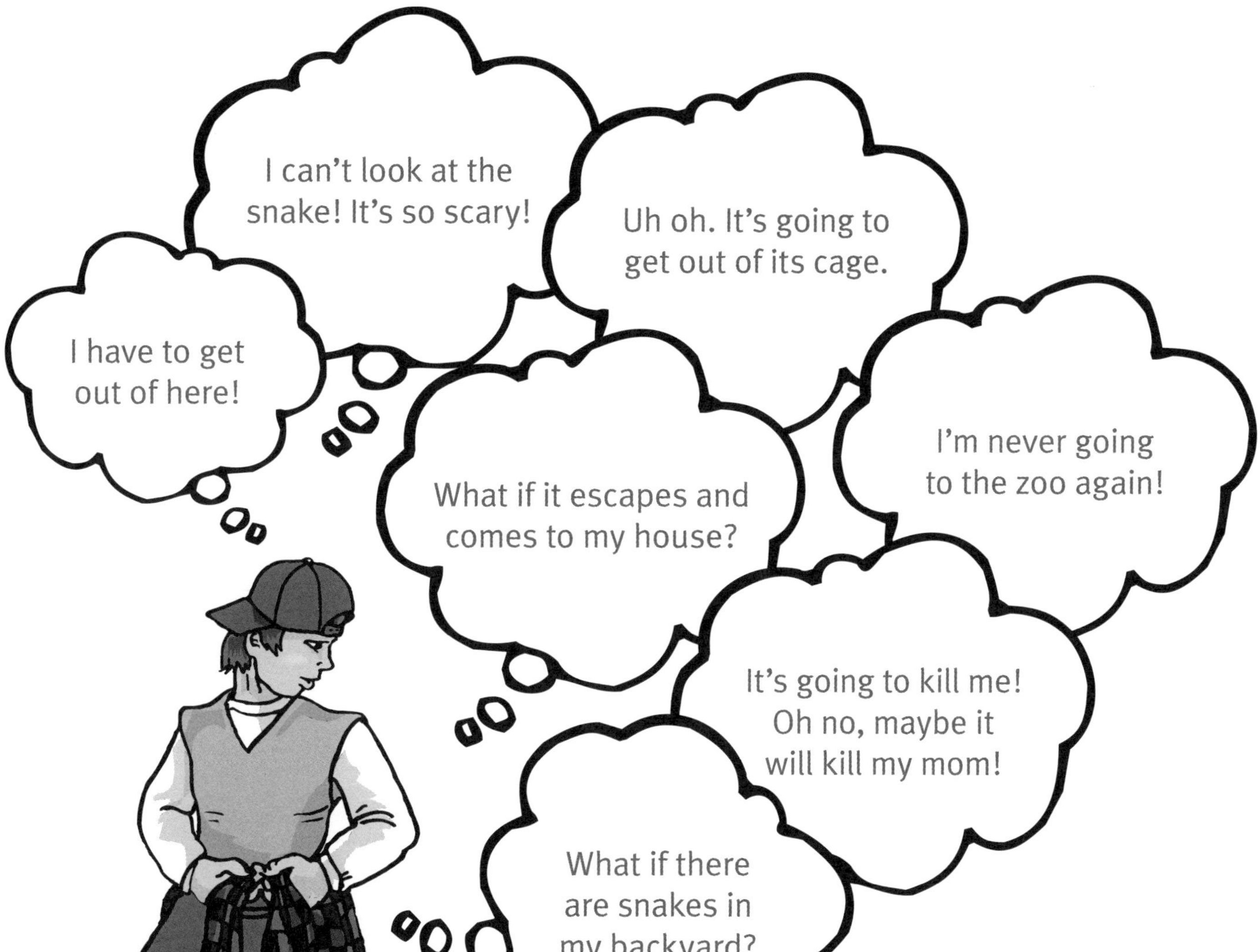

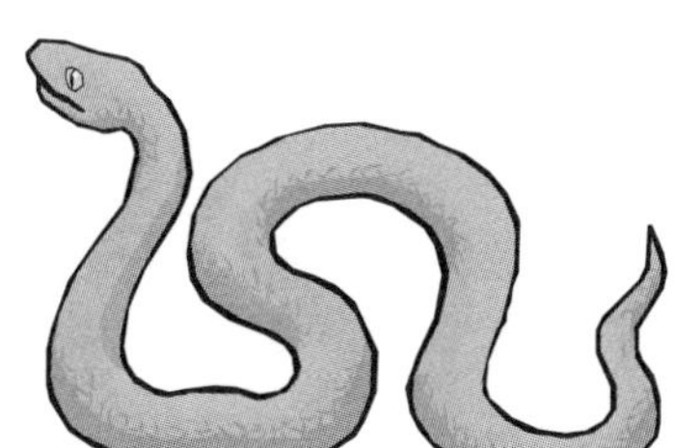

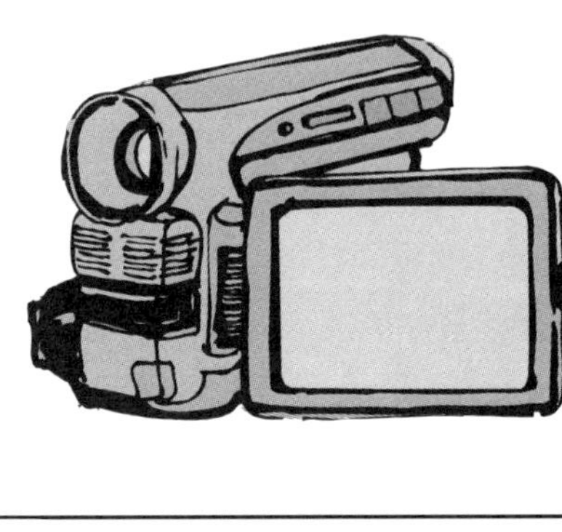

Time John Spends Worrying

John worries about tests, homework, making mistakes, and being late.
How much time do you think he spends worrying?

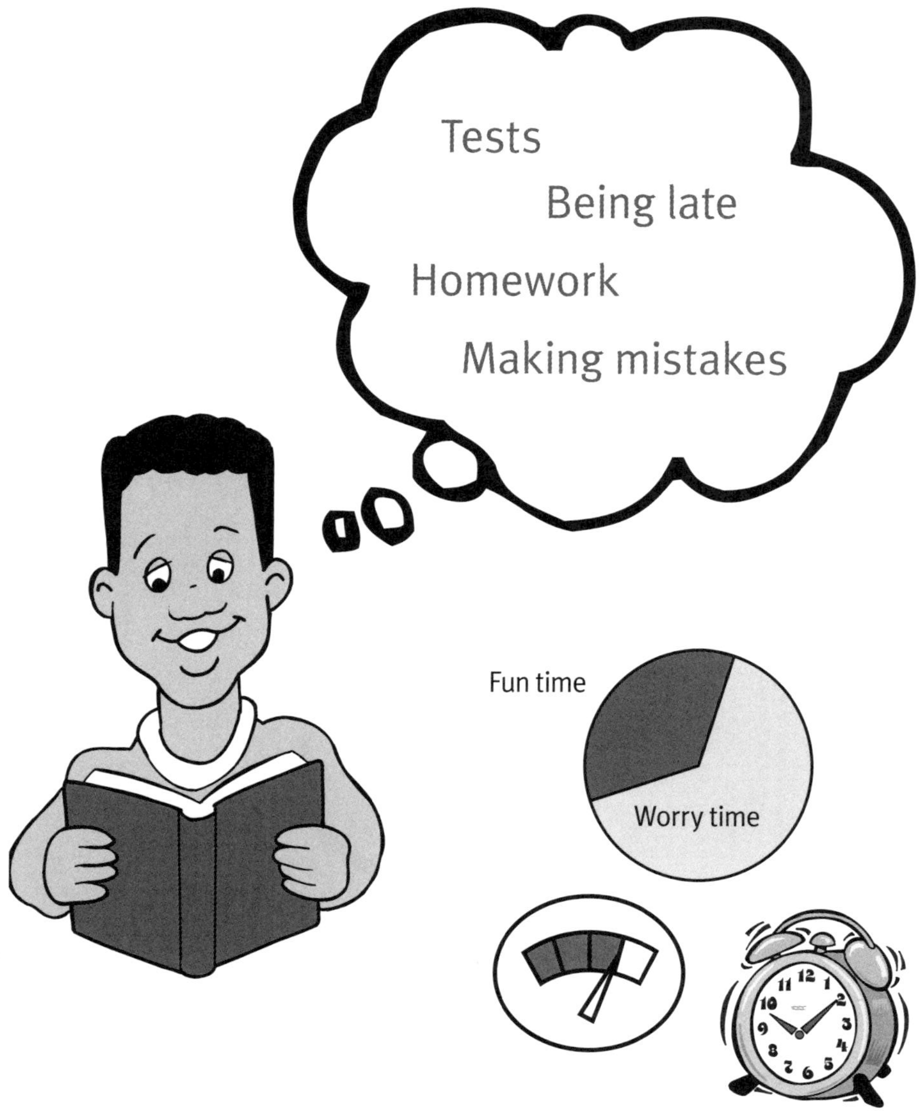

Time John spends worrying

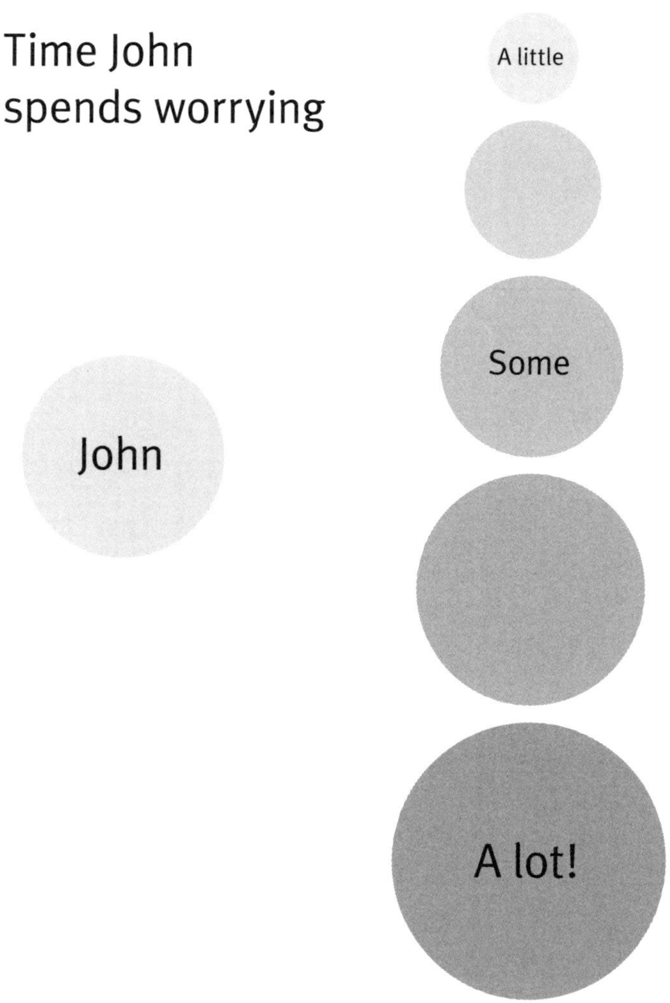

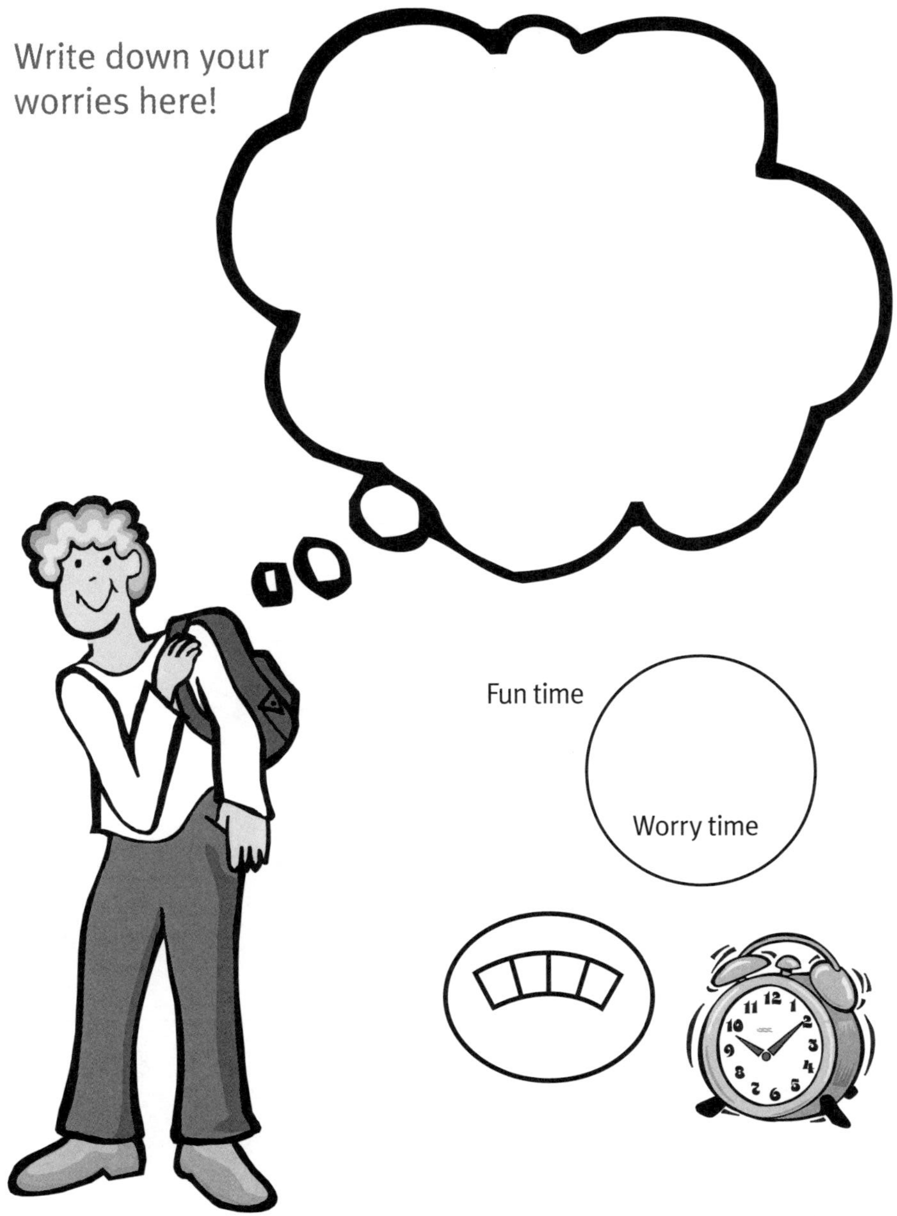

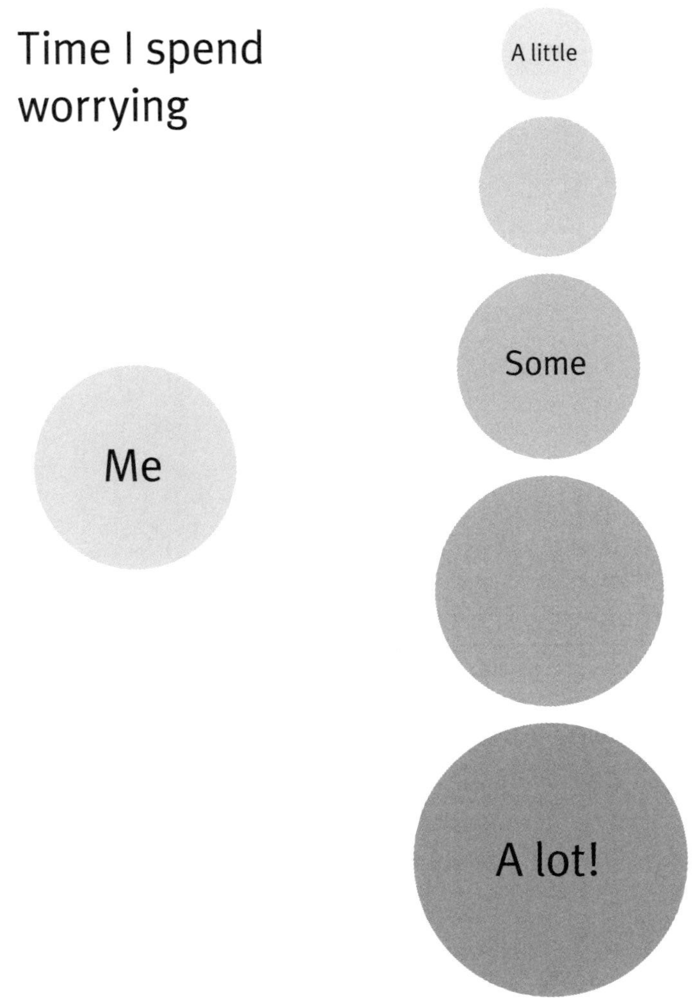

How Much Time Do You Predict You Will Spend Worrying in the Future?

Future worries

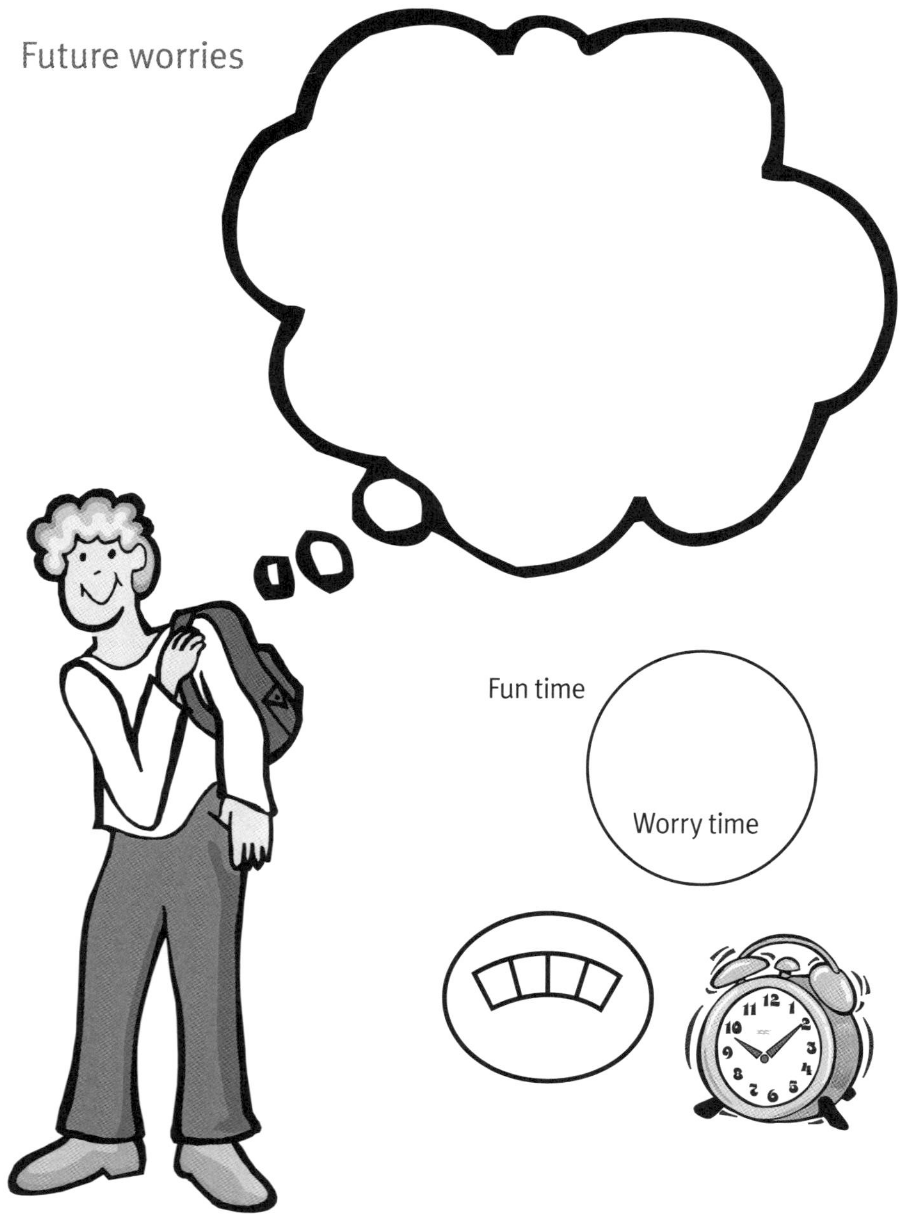

Time I spend worrying

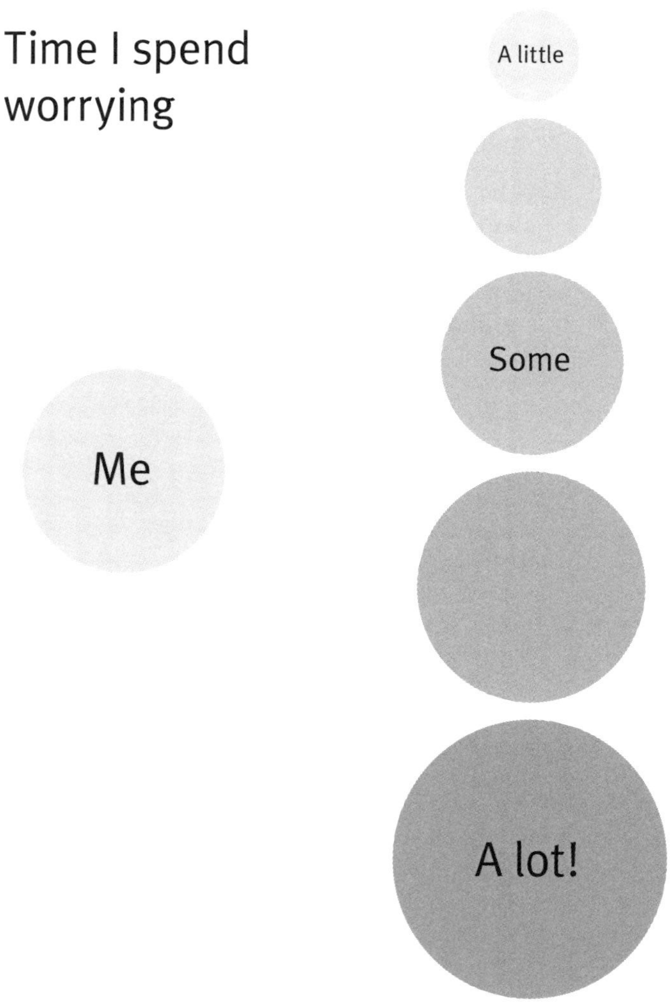

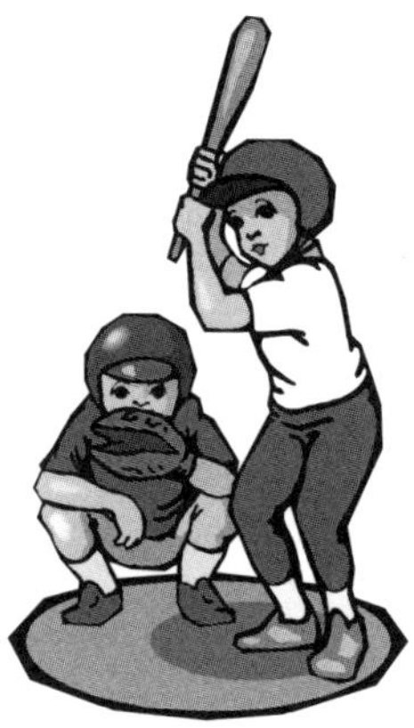 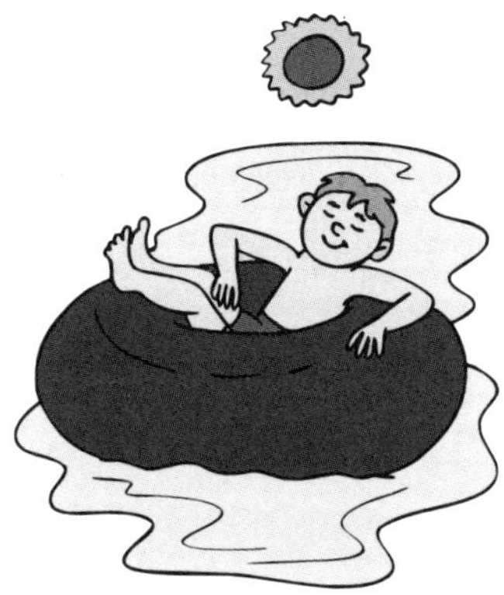 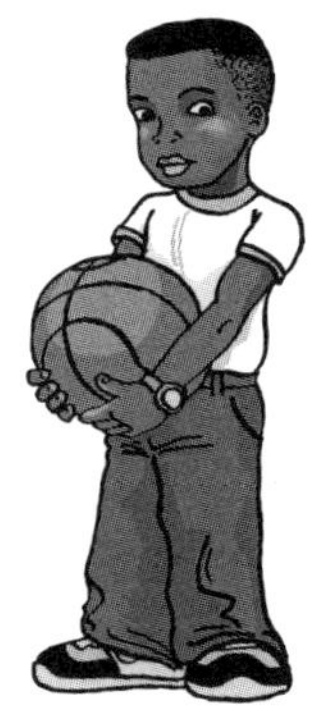

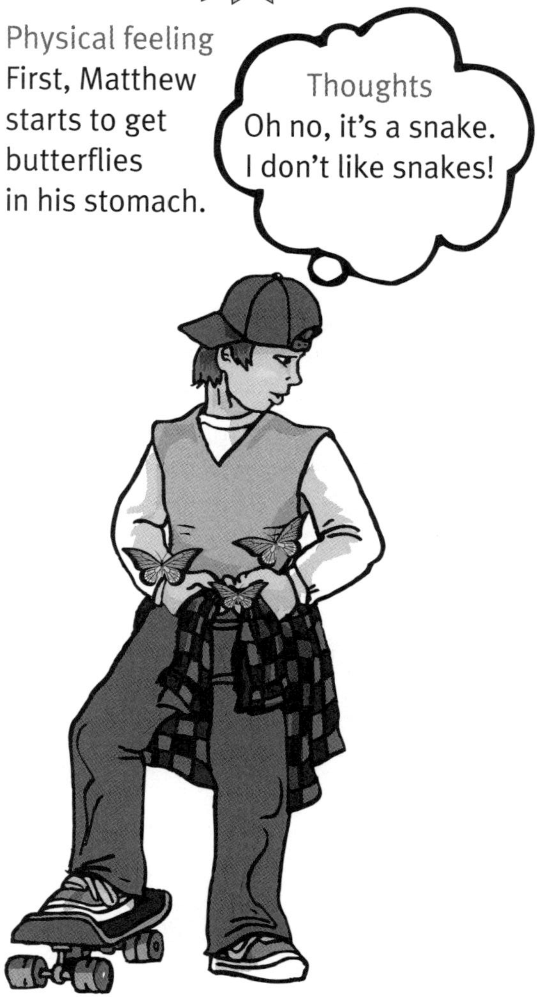

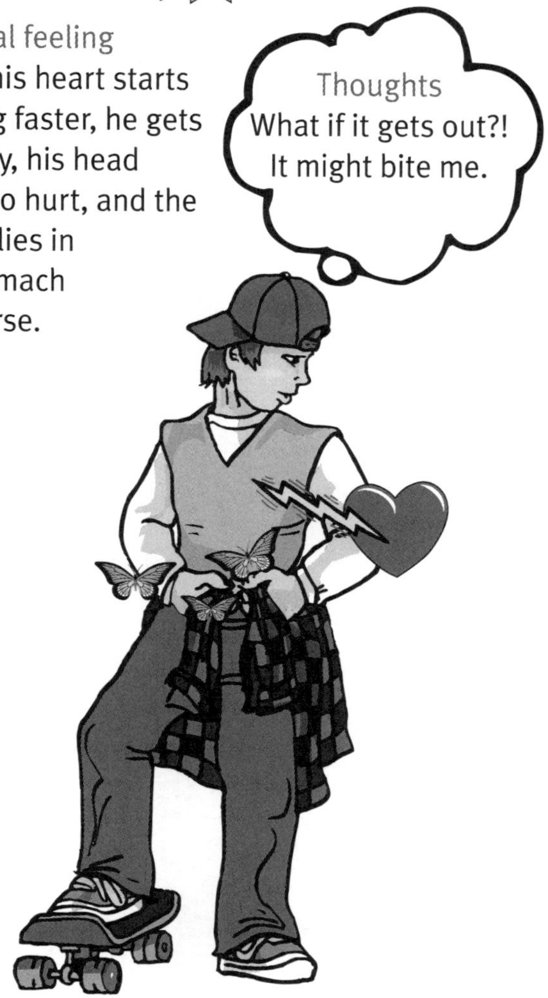

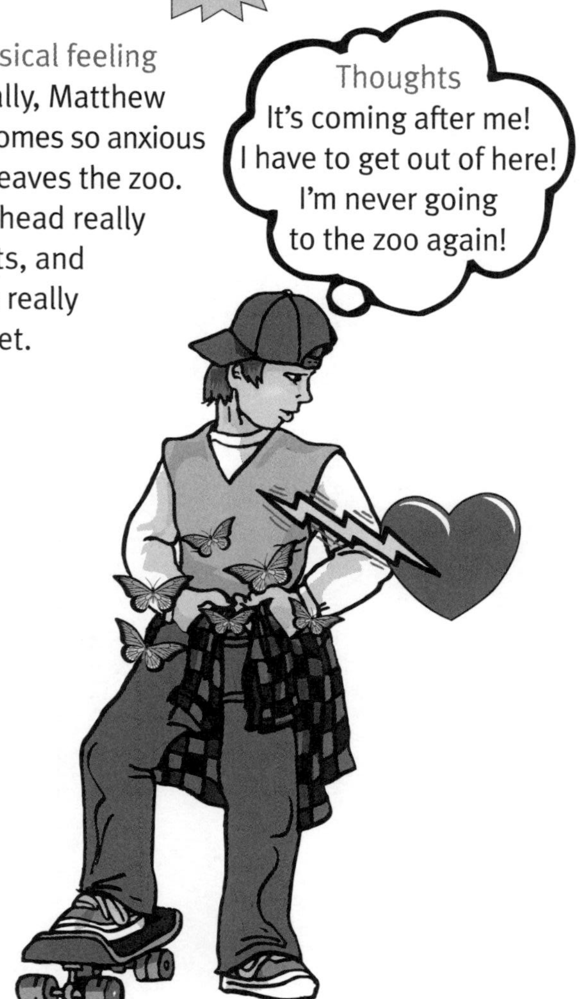

